PREGMANCY

a dad, a little dude, and a due date

PregMANcy Hype

"A laugh-out-loud journey, *PregMANcy* is an honest, real look into the minds and hearts of new fathers. This book isn't just for dads. Moms and any parents-to-be will also love this book because it's packed with stories that hit the raw, funny places where we all really live."
   —Kathy Escobar, author of *Down We Go: Living into the Wild Ways of Jesus*

"*PregMANcy* is a funny, charming, intelligent memoir. With honest hilarity, Christian Piatt's journey toward baby number two will delight and encourage dads and moms of all varieties."
   —Matthew Paul Turner, author of *Churched*

"I have certain expectations when I start a book by Christian Piatt: that it will be hilarious, thoughtful, and a little bit rebellious. *PregMANcy* fulfills those expectations and then some. Piatt is an excellent writer and an even better dad, and this is as engaging a fatherhood book as I've ever read."
   —Jason Boyett, author of *O Me of Little Faith* and the *Pocket Guide* series of books

PREG**MAN**CY

a dad, a little dude, and a due date

By Christian Piatt

CHALICE
PRESS

ST. LOUIS, MISSOURI

Cover design and art: Copyright © 2011 by Mathias Valdez (lastleafprinting.com)

Definition of *Pregmancy* paraphrased from urbandictionary.com.

Interior design: Scribe Inc.

www.chalicepress.com

10 9 8 7 6 5 4 3 2 1   12 13 14 15 16 17

PRINT: 9780827230323 EPUB: 9780827230330 EPDF: 9780827230347

Library of Congress Cataloging-in-Publication Data

Piatt, Christian.
Pregmancy : a dad, a little dude, and a due date / by Christian Piatt.
   p. cm.
  ISBN 978-0-8272-3032-3 (alk. paper)
  1. Fatherhood. 2. Fathers and sons. 3. Mothers. 4. Pregnancy. 5. Piatt, Christian. I. Title.
HQ756.P517 2012
  618.2—dc23
                                                          2012002421

To John "Doc" Edlin, this one's for you

Contents

My Third Trimester

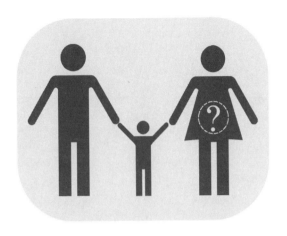

My First Trimester

CHAPTER 1

two fateful words

Mattias: *Daddy, you suck.*

Amy: *Mattias, tell your daddy you're sorry.*

Mattias: *OK. Daddy, I'm sorry you suck.*

—Mattias, 3 years, 3 months

"Screw it."

These two words are what started the baby ball rolling in the Piatt household back in January. After months of counseling, discernment, weepy nights, and sleepless mornings, I submitted, succumbed, and caved in like the roof of a Geo convertible.

I know "screw it" is an ironic choice of words, considering the circumstances. I also think it's sadistically ironic that we men are biologically tuned to love sex so much, yet we're usually the ones who freak out the most about the by-product. I'm a typical male, visually aroused by anything vaguely resembling a boob or a booty. Also, working from home and sharing responsibility with my wife for the daily development of our four-year-old son, Mattias, makes me somewhat abnormal. And it's this shared responsibility, I think, that makes having another kid such a big deal for me.

"I think you take it more seriously than some dads," said a shrink friend of mine who counseled me through some of my initial anxiety when my wife and I first started talking about having more children several months ago. "You know that half of the responsibility of another baby will fall on you, whereas some guys are happy to have more children since they aren't really around that much anyway."

Doc, as I call him, has been both a friend and a physician—and, in many ways, a surrogate father to me—when I've needed him the most. A father of three boys himself, he knows a thing or two about family, and if he's as emotionally and physically available to the rest of his former clients as he is to me, his extended family tree looks like a freaking Chia Pet.

The thing is, even though I love Doc as much as I do anyone else on the planet, he can be kind of a schmuck too. On the one hand, he'll offer up these insightful little gems like this that help validate why I'm so freaked out about expanding our family, and then he'll smile and tell me to stop being such a pansy and just man up.

My wife, Amy, who is nearing her thirty-fourth birthday, is a minister by profession. She's not exactly your typical minister, which should be pretty self-evident, given that she's a woman. We started a church together eight years ago in southern Colorado right after she finished seminary in Texas, just as Mattias turned six months old. We've joked ever since that raising a toddler and starting a church is a whole lot like having twins, but I guess God didn't see that as enough of a challenge for us.

I have my own life outside of the church, which is good since I have yet to receive a paycheck from the church. I help out with everything from music and leadership to outreach, toilet unclogging, landscaping, and whatever else is left unattended to at the end of the day. In some ways I like being a volunteer because it allows me to say "no" more often than if I was paid, though I rarely say "no." It's just nice to know I could if I wanted to. I actually make a living as a writer, which explains how it is that I can at least pretend to have a career, volunteer fifteen or so hours a week at church, and still pitch in my 50 percent toward parenting.

It just seems to me that a full life is a blessing, but only to a point. After that, anything else you pile on just makes you a moron or a masochist, or both. So what I'm left with is a lingering question about why the hell I agreed to this and if it's something I want, or if I'm doing it more or less to keep my wife happy. And at what cost to me?

My wife came down the stairs last Saturday morning with the little pee stick that showed two little red lines indicating that her ticket had been punched. I had no idea that this was coming since I didn't even know she had a secret stash of preggo tests upstairs in the bathroom. The first thing my son wanted to know, of course, was what the pee stick was.

"It's a thermometer," my wife lied, not too eager at that specific moment to explain the implications of what she had only just told me by sticking the pee stick under my nose.

"I wanna try it," he said, pulling it toward his mouth. "Here, take my temperature."

"Not a good idea, monkey," I said, snatching the still-moist stick from Amy's shaky hand. "This one goes in your butt, anyway." That took care of his interest in the pee stick.

She had presented it to me only a few minutes before we took Mattias to play his first soccer game at the YMCA. But the fact that this particular Saturday morning was the day before Mother's Day, and given the fact that, only a few days before, we had talked tentatively about going back on birth control at the end of the month, makes the pee stick incident more than ironic.

So there I sat on the couch, pregnancy test in one hand and coffee cup in the other, pretty much wanting to vomit but trying to smile instead. "Well," I said in a carefully measured tone, giving away nothing, "I guess that means pressure-free sex for the next nine months."

"And my boobs will get huge," said my wife.

"Yeah, there is that, I guess." Now I was giving my feelings away.

"It's kind of like cheating," she said after a pause, "but with me, attached to someone else's boobs."

"Thanks," I sighed, "but you don't have to sell me."

There was a long, pregnant silence.

"Guess we ought to get ready to go to the soccer game," she said, holding herself up along the back of the couch.

"Guess so." I rolled off the edge of the couch and to my feet. "The Mighty Giraffes won't wait forever." As I helped Mattias get his shin guards on and double-knot his soccer shoes, I felt for Amy, knowing she was hoping for more excitement from me, but I couldn't help but imagine trying to do it with a little slobbering machine under one arm. There are plenty of things that stress me out about the idea of having another baby, but the messiness of it all is right up there. I'm not exactly a neat freak, but I do like things a certain way. Amy can tell you that surprises and I are not good friends, which will give you some idea about how I felt toward the telltale pee stick. My Blackberry and I are good friends because it's the informational equivalent of heroin in my pocket at all times, but also because it reminds me of everything in my life that is going to happen, fifteen minutes before it does.

Babies, on the other hand, are unpredictable. I'll talk about this more later, but I'm not the greatest at handling this. I have gotten better about managing chaos in the last few years. Family, after all, is a choice I have made. It hasn't been forced upon me, and I wouldn't give it up for anything else in the world. But it's messy, unpredictable, and stressful as hell. It doesn't help that my son—though brilliant, funny, and infinitely charming—has a wild and independent streak a mile long. One of the reassurances that some advisors and friends have offered is that the odds of having another child as strong-willed as Mattias is statistically improbable, but my thinking is that Mattias plus anything else—even a slightly animated sack of sweet potatoes—may be more than I can handle.

As we headed out the door to the soccer field, I was already telling myself that worrying about it wasn't going to get me anywhere.

It's coming whether I'm ready or not.

At least I have about eight more months to get used to the idea, I thought. Maybe I'll pour my thoughts out onto the page, administer some self-service therapy.

But right now, I'm pretty much back to where I started:

Screw it.

CHAPTER 2

anticontraception

It smells like daddy in here. It smells like poop.

—Mattias, 2 years, 11 months

This time around, I have learned two things for sure about the baby-making process:

1. The rhythm method is a joke.
2. Wine is the ultimate anticontraceptive.

I know the day, if not the minute, when this little experiment was kicked off. Amy and I had committed to trying to have a date night once a week after realizing we had failed to spend any real, quality adult time together in about a month and a half. This may seem hard to imagine given that we both work from home, but I've come to believe that even though I imagined we would spend more time together, in some ways we end up with less.

Now if you want to be a nerd about it and actually calculate the hours in a day when we're within eyeshot of each other, yeah, we see each other plenty. And it's not that we live into the old cliché about familiarity breeding contempt; although it certainly breeds something, doesn't it, class?

Anyway, the point is that sometimes being around each other so much makes you almost invisible to one another. It's kind of like the way you look at your favorite sofa, although Amy will probably kill me for comparing her to a piece of furniture. You sit on the thing every single day, but how often do you really take time to notice it? Of course, I don't spend a lot of time sitting on Amy, but there are days when we'll be around each other pretty much every single hour, day and night, awake and asleep.

We get teased down at our local coffee shop, where we like to work a couple of days a week, because we've been known to set up our laptops back-to-back so they're just barely touching but also so we can hardly see each other.

"Aww, isn't that cute," someone will quip. "It's almost like they're holding hands." Truth is, we may share a file now and then, make a comment about something we're reading, or check our calendars for conflicting events, but we can also just as easily sit at the same table for hours and not say a damn thing to each other.

I won't say that I'd have our lives set up any other way if I had the choice. It's not as if I'd wish I had a cubicle to stuff myself into every day so I'd really know what I was missing. On the contrary, there are those mornings when the temperature is just right and neither of us is too buried with work and we'll pack up the computers and go for a walk or hit the thrift stores. There are the afternoons spent at the park with Mattias, chasing ducks and filling our shoes with sand, but I guess when I imagined working from home, I expected to end up doing a lot more of that than I actually do.

The reality is that we don't work any less because we are on our own schedules. In some ways, we end up doing more because there is no one there to tell us to go home, unplug, and get a real life. My laptop stays running about three feet from my spot on the couch most every minute of every day I'm awake. Amy has joked about being jealous of the time I spend with my Toshiba, but she's only halfway kidding.

As for Amy, a minister never really takes off from work. The next phone call might be a life-or-death crisis, and people aren't really forward-thinking enough about when they die to plan around your date nights. A church member is just as likely to have a stroke at 3 a.m. on Friday as they are to call with news of a new job right in the middle of lunch. Your availability is part of what people are paying for in giving a minister a full-time salary. Just what is meant by "full time" isn't always exactly clear, but it has something to do with being available when people need you, which is anytime, anywhere.

So we both have careers that allow us, in some ways, to be more present to one another and, in other ways, to always have one half of our brain committed to something else.

Back to date night. This particular Friday night, we had arranged for a babysitter to come take care of Mattias and made plans to visit our favorite restaurant in town. In Pueblo, Colorado, where we live, you basically have two choices when it comes to dining anywhere other than in a chain restaurant, so you'd better like Mexican or Italian food. Turns out, fortunately for us, that we like both.

On the rare occasions when we have the chance to share a whole night with each other, it's also a special treat to share a bottle of our favorite Chianti. The only thing I love more than homemade Italian food with a glass of Chianti is sharing the two with a hot chick. As a man who has been married nearly eight years—and who would like to shoot for many more to come—I would never suggest that there's a single minute of any day when my wife is not attractive, but this night was one of those nights that provided extra opportunity for me to reflect on my spouse's natural beauty.

It doesn't take a genius to see where this night ended up, but I should back up and address the first point about how much the rhythm method sucks. This so-called contraception method involves mapping out your partner's menstrual cycles so you know which days of the month are safer than others to have sex without protection. And though we're Protestants, we knew it was the favored strategy for horny Catholics and Mormons who, by mandate of their faith, are not allowed to use condoms or other birth control, but who still like to doink as much as others.

Amy had stopped taking her pill back in January following the "screw it" conversation. For a few months, I wavered between moderate acceptance and near impotence-inducing anxiety about the realization that any amorous encounter could have a much bigger payoff than the average romp. In fact, my own discomfort with the pressure got to be so bad that we had just had a conversation a couple of weeks prior about exploring other methods of birth control, since it's not a good idea for a woman to go on and off the pill very often.

In an effort to help me feel better, Amy had discreetly printed out a calendar of her projected ovulation times, complete with the most fertile days highlighted in yellow so you knew either to target them or avoid them, depending on your intentions. I guess the combination of knowing, based on this piece of paper, that she should not have been ovulating, combined with the emboldening effect of a half a bottle of wine, made me feel like kicking things up a notch once we got home. Sounded like a great idea to me.

"You know what?" I said, as we lay together on the couch after the babysitter drove herself home, "We really should have sex, don't you think?"

Another thing I truly love about my wife is that she never takes a roundabout invitation to sex as a rhetorical question. She was practically undressed before I got "don't you think" out of my mouth. And don't get me wrong, it was the perfect end to our first date night in more than a month.

Do I think Amy manipulated her ovulation calendar on purpose in order to lull me into sleeping with her? Of course not. That's just not the kind of relationship we have. Sure, go ahead and be cynical if you want, but as stressed out as I may be about having another baby, there's not a single part of me that thinks Amy did this to me. I have control over my own body parts, where they go and what they do. Now I may have a little worse judgment after three glasses of Chianti, but I still can't blame that on anyone but myself.

Still, once this pregnancy and delivery is all over, someone in the Piatt household is getting snipped. I've happily offered my little fellas up for a vasectomy, but if things go the way they did with Mattias, Amy may end up in the operating room. If they have to open her up to get this one out, they might as well take care of the plumbing in a two-for-one deal. It's not like I'm excited about anyone having a scalpel that close to my balls anyway, but since she has to go through the agony of childbirth, I figure this is my opportunity to "pitch in."

Luckily, I have a little while before I have to make my contribution to our family planning. But while she's basking in the warm glow of imminent motherhood for the second time, I intend to use my sacrifice of remaining a fully functioning procreator for whatever points that may earn me.

And no matter what happens, this is the last time a bottle of wine and some stupid calendar we get off the Internet will be the cornerstones of our family planning.

CHAPTER 3

what could go wrong?

Don't ever kill me, OK? Killing me is not safe.

—Mattias, 3 years, 0 months

"What's your greatest fear about having another baby?"

I don't think Amy was just goading me when she asked me this back in the early stages of impending double fatherhood, but she knows we're both pretty good worriers (though I'd argue she's better at it than I am, and since I'm the one writing this book, we'll assume she'd agree with me).

Talk about an open invitation to worry! I don't spend a lot of energy worrying about day-to-day matters; I'm more of a saver. But when something comes along that's really worth worrying about, you can bet I'll draw down that worry account a bit.

After Amy asked me the fateful question, I started compiling a mental list. I figure I'll lay out at least my top ten here for your edification, or at least for simple amusement:

#10. We could have twins: I can't base this on any real facts, but it seems I've read or heard or seen somewhere the older people are, the greater chance they have of multiple births. I suppose I could go look this up and settle it in my own mind one way or the other, but it's a lot more fun to worry about it. Twins don't run in the bloodlines on either side of the family, but that's all the more reason to worry about it, right? Aren't we probably due?

Imagining a baby in each arm is just about enough to make me pass out. And that doesn't even begin to touch the effect it would have on my wife, who plans to breastfeed as long as she can. Hell, I'd never see those puppies again. I'll be lucky if they don't fall off, right on to the floor, by the time the twin suckers are done with them.

#9. He/she could end up like me: All things considered, I think I have an amazing life, but it hasn't been all wine and roses getting to this point. I may tell you more about the summer I spent in lockdown at a psychiatric hospital, and the years I mixed my antianxiety meds with beer and weed, but suffice it to say, for the sake of my worry list, there are significant parts of myself that I have no interest in passing on to my progeny.

It's really too early to know if Mattias will struggle with some of the same problems that I had—that I still have—but I am pretty sure that if he does, I can cover therapy for one kid. Add another one to the mix and, considering my history, it seems a little bit like playing psychological Russian roulette.

#8. He/she could end up like any number of our relatives: I know I run the risk of bruising some egos with this statement, but most people in my family, or Amy's family, will readily admit that we have a plenitude of addicts, going back many generations. My dad and I haven't spoken in more than two years due to problems revolving around addiction and related issues. His father started most mornings with a cocktail, and he found his mother—my great-grandmother—in the garage of their house after she had shot herself.

My grandmother on my mom's side has been known to rely heavily on an exotic combination of prescription pain meds and muscle relaxers and was prone to washing them down with some white zinfandel, at least back before she and my grandfather moved into my mom's house. I'll leave Amy to spill her own beans, but more than a handful of her immediate relatives have gratefully found a new life in recovery, while others arguably still actively practice self-destructive behavior.

I don't want to sound like I'm knocking addicts; on the contrary, Amy and I tend to love them. In fact, those who have struggled with addiction and lived to tell about it often are the most charming, funny, and interesting people I know. On the other hand, that addiction is always there, just under the surface, and is most likely to rear its head when ignored or minimized.

We go to great lengths to teach Mattias solid judgment, self-care, moderation, and recognizing the difference between needs and wants. But every now and then, I see these obsessive little glimmers in his personality that make me wonder if he has that same unscratchable itch. To witness a child succumb to the ravages of addiction is about the worst fate I can imagine, and not unlike the whole depression and anxiety I have, it seems a bit like we're tempting fate with another one.

#7. *We can't afford it:* I know, whoever has room in their budget for another kid? Of course, when priorities present themselves like this you find a way, but the financial stress can be a killer. Maybe we ought to move, sell a car, or donate plasma. If being a sperm donor was a cash cow industry, I might go that route since I'm obviously not planning to use any of my man-juice for my own purposes anymore.

This doesn't even begin to take care of birth-related expenses. With both of us being self-employed, we have crappy insurance, to put it mildly. We have a $5,000 annual deductible and, oh, did I mention maternity isn't covered? Brilliant.

#6. *Birth defects:* If I'm going to put my worries out there, I can't leave this one out. I'm going to be thirty-seven years old, after all, by the time this baby arrives, and Amy will be thirty four. Though we're not technically considered to fall in the highest-risk age brackets yet, we're not that far from it. And it doesn't help that, a few months ago, some close friends of ours gave birth to a daughter with Down's syndrome. Like them, we would love the kid no matter what and, also like them, we'd find the good in the unexpected. But for now, before we know any better, all I end up doing is worrying about it.

I know that part of this concern comes from my career before I started working with nonprofits, back when I worked in clinics for kids with learning disabilities. I saw kids with everything from mild dyslexia to autism, cerebral palsy, and worse. There was one family in particular that I remember who had three of the sweetest kids I'd ever met in my life. The thing is, all three had an incredibly rare disease that not only affected their development but also was expected to prove fatal for all of them before they graduated high school. Nevertheless, the parents insisted on trying to provide every opportunity to help their children's lives be as normal as possible, and I felt blessed to be a part of those hopeful moments. But every day they didn't make it to the clinic because the buildup of fluid in their brains caused migraines or made them lose feelings in their limbs; it tore me up inside

It was all I could do to hold it together for those three little guys, and they weren't even my kids. What the hell will I do if I have one of my own?

#5. *Delivery complications:* Amy was a real trooper when Mattias was born, but nothing about it was easy. Actually he and I had eerily similar experiences making our way into the world. We both were exactly the same length and weight, we both were faced the wrong way, and both of us were finally delivered by cesarian section, after putting our moms through hours of hardcore labor.

The story I've heard is that my delivery was a big part of why my folks decided not to have any more children. Before that, they planned on having more but it was too much to deal with. And let me tell you that I can sympathize. I was in the room both when Amy tried to deliver naturally, and when they cut her wide open and yanked the little peanut out, his face was blue from a lack of oxygen and his umbilical cord wrapped twice around his neck. Though I've never experienced such awe and joy in my life, I also have no desire to relive that sort of terrifying vulnerability.

#4. Postpartum: We didn't recognize it as such for almost a year, but Amy suffered from pretty severe postpartum depression after Mattias was born. In a phrase, it sucked. I also happened to be running for local political office at the time, which added stress to the situation, but I didn't know what the hell was going on. It was our first time, after all, and no one really warned us about what to do if your wife has quasi-psychotic images of herself pushing your baby down the stairs. She was so worried she was going crazy that she didn't tell anyone for fear that they might take Mattias away from her. So instead, she tried to manage it, quite unsuccessfully, on her own for nearly twelve months.

The breaking point finally came one night when we were lying in bed and I laid it all out. I knew something was really wrong, but I had no idea what it was. I could feel her withdrawing farther away from me every day, and I felt like I couldn't do anything about it. I'd asked her to get into therapy or to talk to her physician, but again, she was worried they'd stamp her forehead with "LOONEY" in big, red letters and cart her off on a gurney. One way or another, though, something had to change. As much as it broke my heart to say it, I finally gave her an ultimatum. I told her that if she didn't get help, I wasn't sure we'd make it as a family.

It was only a matter of weeks after that before things started getting notably better. She got on some good antidepressants and hit the shrink's couch for several months. But I think the greatest healing came from knowing that not only was postpartum depression normal but it was treatable. This time around, we already have plans for proactive intervention to reduce the likelihood of a recurrence, but anyone who's been through a major car wreck or similar traumatic event can tell you that no number of seatbelts or airbags will really ever make you feel as safe as you'd like again.

#3. We'll forget how to be married: I already mentioned in the first chapter about how we struggle to put time aside just for us. Our plan to have a weekly date night has been met with mixed results at best, but not for lack of trying. Every time we do spend an evening or some other

real intentional time together, it helps me remember why I married Amy in the first place and why I still love her. Without that, it's way too easy to slip into survival mode and look at each other more as parents or business partners rather than as lovers.

With only a few family members in town, and the fact that Mattias doesn't exactly offer an autopilot sort of babysitting gig, it's already a challenge to find good babysitters. I'm sure that adding another body to the formula will not make that search any easier.

Of course, date nights are only part of the larger issue. It's all too easy for parents to fall into "survival mode," pouring all their energy into being good parents until there's nothing left. But as plenty of us born in the last forty years can attest, divorces mess kids up, no matter how good of a parent you are.

#2. She'll want another one: Amy says she understands that I have no interest in more kids after this, and that even number two is stretching my sanity a bit, nearly eight months out. But here's the thing: I think it's plenty easy for a woman to say she doesn't want another baby while she's pregnant. That's a little bit like congratulating yourself for turning down a chocolate chip cookie while you're devouring a cake. The real test will be once the hormones regulate themselves and the whole baby amnesia kicks in, so that she forgets what a bitch labor is and how much of a drag it is not to sleep for an entire year straight.

It's not that I don't believe her when she says she doesn't want another one. It's just that not wanting one right now isn't really the same as not wanting another one for the rest of our lives.

#1. We lose it: For at least another month and a half, there's a pretty high risk of miscarriage, and our odds aren't helped by Amy being in her midthirties. Though a miscarriage isn't the end of the world, I'm pretty sure I'm not going to want to step back into the batter's box if it happens. If this possibility becomes reality, we'll have the loss itself to deal with compounded by the fact that she will still likely want a baby. But given that scenario, I'm pretty sure I'll only dig my heels in deeper, which could lead to who-knows-what kind of resentment and weirdness between us.

"The biggest sadness I think I have for you about all of this," Doc said to me, "is that you're not jumping up and down with joy."

He's right; I'm not. I'm trying to come to terms with it, but joy would not be an accurate description of my state of mind right now. It's a shame to think about looking back later and regretting not being more present and joyful about a new life coming into our family, but all these damn hang-ups keep getting in the way. Doc knows this. After all, he knows me as well as, or better than, anyone.

"Are you considering termination?" he asked, in his best clinical, matter-of-fact tone.

"What?" It wasn't that I didn't hear him, but I was kind of shocked that he would even ask me such a question. It actually kind of pissed me off. Now that I've gotten some emotional distance from the call, I think he knew exactly what he was doing. He knew that no matter how freaked out I was about this, I'd never, ever consider an abortion. Either that or he doesn't know me nearly as well as I thought he did.

Basically, he's presenting me with an absurd alternative to help me get things into perspective. Of course I'm going to follow through. Of course I'll love this kid no matter what, regardless of how many heads it has or if we're living on food stamps to make ends meet. So what's the solution? The raw, primitive guy center in my brain says the only thing to do is to get the hell over it.

Buddhists have another, possibly more philosophical way of putting it. They have a saying that's become a favorite of mine, which goes something like this:

"If there's a problem and there's something you can do about it, then don't worry about it. If there's a problem and there's nothing you can do about it, don't worry about it either."

Nice enough to say, but how many Buddhist monks have had to worry about their wives dying in the delivery room, leaving them with a baby in each hand and no clue how to raise them without help? Sure it's irrational, but fear is powerful, whether it has much of a basis in reality or not.

Worry may not fix a thing, but on occasion it can help distract you from your real problems. It would be nice if our issues were as easy to spot as the monster we all used to imagine lived in the closet or under the bed. But sometimes they take a much more subtle form. Big, yellow eyes and gnashing teeth are well and good for dramatic effect, but in the real world nothing is more terrifying than the prospect of losing what you love most, like a child.

That kind of fear is way more potent than any of the fantasy crap. It happens every day. That fear is the steep price of love.

CHAPTER 4

too smart

Christian: *Mattias, you did a really good job playing the tambourine.*

Mattias: *I know, but I peed my pants.*

—Mattias, 3 years, 3 months

One of the bigger worries I left off the list is that my kid is smart. Most parents think their kids are smart, and some of them are right. But my recognition of my son's intelligence really is a statement of observation and not bragging about him.

By eighteen months, Mattias knew his letters, and by shortly after his third birthday, he started to read. He does double-digit arithmetic in his head at age four, and his memory has some sort of internal hermetic seal on it that, from what I can tell, never lets anything back out once it enters. We haven't had him tested, and for the foreseeable future, we have no reason to. He's happy in preschool, and he still has a whole lot to learn about taking turns, sharing, using kind words, and even paying enough attention to his body not to piss himself when he's overly excited about a game with friends.

To say that Mattias is verbal is a dramatic understatement. He started talking at a year old and hasn't shut up ever since. He's precociously charming and challenging, intellectually curious and occasionally maddening. However, none of this touches the most mind-blowing moment Amy and I had recently experienced with him. Amy was in the kitchen, heating up some chicken noodle soup in the microwave for his lunch, and Mattias trailed close behind her as she brought it in to the living room table.

"The microwave makes a 'G,' you know," he said as he slurped noodles off his chin. I thought he was talking about the food somehow, as I'm pretty used to weird four-year-old nonsequiturs by now.

"A 'G,' huh?" I said, not even looking up from my computer.

"Yep, a 'G,'" he started humming a note, and that's when I realized he was talking about that the frequency that the microwave motor was making. I decided I'd check him against the piano, so I went over and tapped out a 'G.' He was within a quarter-step, between G and G sharp.

"Wow, buddy. That was pretty close. Good job."

"No, dad," Mattias rolled his eyes. "it *is* a 'G.'" He never lacks for confidence, even when he's amazingly wrong, but he was so sure of himself, I figured I'd double-check against his keyboard.

Turns out it's been a while since we've had our piano tuned. It's about a quarter-step out of whack.

I took him to his keyboard and played notes without letting him look at what I was playing. He nailed every one: sharps, flats, the whole works. Then I played two- and three-note chords, and he could tell me all of those notes. For the final test, I played six- to eight-note sequences, all in a row, and he rattled off the notes as if it was so obvious any idiot should know it.

"Here dad," he pulled the keyboard onto his lap, "let me try." He started plunking out a few notes and waiting for my answers. I got a few of them, leaning on half a dozen years of music school and ear training, along with a decent sense of pitch memory. But since I taught Mattias the notes—keeping in mind he's only four years old—he has never once misidentified a note he's heard.

Now his new hobby is telling me what key every song he hears on the radio is in. He also likes to take the songs he learns at school and rearrange them with a three-four swing or a bossa nova beat. It's a phenomenal thing to observe, and it definitely makes you realize you're witnessing something over which you have little or no control, let alone any understanding.

You can improve your pitch through years of ear training and music practice, but there are those rare few who are just born with it. To Mattias, it doesn't make any sense that anyone else wouldn't be able to just know what the notes are that they hear. He looks at me like I'm some kind of moron, and I've had years of training. I can only imagine how he would come across to someone who didn't know what he was talking about.

I remember the feeling I had when I first realized he had what experts call absolute, or perfect, pitch. I was at once exhilarated, a little freaked out, and admittedly a little jealous. Imagine you studied a language your whole life, and just as you're starting to really feel like you're fluent, a kindergartener walks into the same class and, after the first lesson, comes out speaking better than you. To add to the insult, they look at you like some kind of tool for not being able to keep up.

Now imagine that's your kid looking at you and you're the tool.

It would be nice to be responsible for his musical skill, but all I did was expose him to music, get him some instruments, and teach him the notes. The rest was just in there. My excitement came from the realization that he can probably accomplish incredible things if he decides to pursue music with some focus. At four years old, though, music should be fun, so there's not a lot we're going to do about it except try to find him a teacher who can help stretch him a bit, but who recognizes that the joy of music is more important than getting him out on the tour circuit.

It's also a little overwhelming to know that your kid has an ability that you will never be able to equal. In most cases, we have at least a handful of years within which to teach our children what we know, which also tilts the balance of power in our favor. Some of us may not want to admit it, but it's an awesome ego boost to have a little person look at you with that wide-eyed stare, like you simply must know pretty much every single thing in the world. But if your preschooler already can do something better than you, especially if you've been working at it your whole life, face it, you're pretty much screwed.

Even though he's my son, it's hard to see someone get handed something I have worked really hard for. This is a fruitless way to spend energy since, first of all, I'd never wish anything less for him and, second, I have the skills that I have and that needs to be good enough. Instead of focusing on what I lack, which is much easier than focusing on discipline, I can find plenty of excuses for not doing more with where I am in life. *Oh, if only I had what she had, or looked like he did, or was born into his family, then I'd be* (fill in the blank).

We always compare ourselves to others, that's part of our human makeup. But when we become beholden to that sort of external sense of worth, whether it's living vicariously through our children's lives, or comparing ourselves to them or the guy next door, we're focusing on wishes rather than reality, and we're pretty well doomed to be unsatisfied with wherever we are, regardless of what we have.

How is it that a little kid who can barely wipe his own butt has the power to raise all of this inside of me? He has no idea, which is probably best, because if he knew what a mess I was, God knows what that would do to his worldview. And how will it be with a second kid, especially with

Mattias around to dispel any notion that his parents are any less than dumbasses, making it up as we go along?

To some degree, kids need to see their parents as perfect so they feel sufficiently safe during their most vulnerable years. The problem is when we start believing in the same illusion. I think one reason teenagers start to act like their parents are idiots is because they're starting to come to terms with the idea that those parents they've held on a pedestal for so long actually are flawed, just like the rest of the world. So as tempting as it is to feed into the idea that we're flawless, we offer our kids more when we show them we're human, capable of fault, but also worth loving and respecting regardless.

So the tricky balance for me is giving Mattias the love and support he needs, while also earning his respect. I don't have to be as good as he is at any age, and the best way he'll understand this is if we keep our admiration for his gifts separate from our love for him as a human being. It's harder to do than to say, though. I mean, how easy is it to go over and give your boy a hug after he's done something brilliant? And it's not that hugging him is wrong in that case, but if that's the only time he sees love expressed, then he's going to draw an imaginary line between the two and draw the conclusion that to be loved he has to be a little prodigy.

And how do you balance it with two kids? How can you possibly keep from comparing them, or keep the world from comparing them? Inevitably one will be both better and worse than the other at any number of things, and vice versa. What if the next kid's gifts are seen as a little less remarkable than Mattias's obvious talents? And then of course there's the concern that they won't fully live into their potential. So now we're not only doubling the challenge of building up healthy identities for two other separate human beings; it actually almost seems like a setup for number two to have to follow in Mattias's footsteps.

This is the kind of thing that would keep me up at night when Amy wanted another baby, with the little voice in the back of my head telling me over and over to quit while I'm ahead.

This whole matter of ability, affection, and the connection between the two was a point of confusion in my family of origin. It's a little awkward to talk about yourself in what could be interpreted as a self-congratulatory way, but it's meant to make a point. My mom loves to recall the stories of me as a toddler, much like Mattias, when I learned my letters at sixteen months, started spelling at about the same age as he, and so on. I got bored in public school about halfway through first grade, and the school administrators explained to my parents that they were running out of material to keep me busy. When my folks suggested they give me second-grade work, they explained that they had, and that they meant they were running out of any elementary school materials to occupy me.

That's when they took me in to get me tested. The doctors didn't tell my parents exact numbers or anything, but the next thing I knew I was in private schools where, all of a sudden, they expected me to work and I wasn't the smartest kid in the class. After the initial shock, I got used to it and actually came to enjoy it, but my dad got a little bit obsessed with IQs after that. My mom talks about how he often talked about getting himself tested, and he even did a mini-MENSA test from a magazine one time. When he scored very well, he tossed it over to my mom as a sort of challenge. The fact that she narrowly beat him didn't go over too well. I was too young to take it, but he had T-shirts reflecting their scores and, indicating that, had I been able to take it, I'd probably have waxed both of them. You could interpret this as family pride, but that seems a weird thing to advertise.

There were a number of other examples like this, but it was clear that the older I got, the more awkwardness there became between me and my dad about our intellects. A silent low-level competition, always just below the surface. It didn't help when I rebelled, dropping out of an elite private school to finish my high school years at a public magnet school for music. Nor were they thrilled when I passed on a chance to attend Duke in favor of the music school up the road at the University of North Texas. I'm sure some of my choices by that point were brazen rebellion, but those were also some of the happiest years of my life. What will be hard is when I have "X" plans for my kids and they choose "Y," either because they've been raised to think for themselves or, maybe just as likely, they do it just to get a rise out of their parents.

As a parent, you want to see your kids make the most of the opportunities they have. However, how that plays out is only partly under our control. I think it's also all right to give ourselves permission to be human beings, whether that means trying too hard to be perfect, longing for what others have, pushing a little too hard, or simply loving inconsistently sometimes. Amy and I joke that our kids will have one of two choices when they graduate high school: college or therapy. We're saving enough for one or the other, but if they are too screwed up to go on to college without seeing a shrink, they better get some frigging scholarships.

It's guaranteed that we'll screw our kids up to some degree, and it's also a reality that most of them will live through it, regardless of what kind of a job we do. If I've learned anything so far, it can be summed up in these three rules for parenting:

1. Think of yourself as a witness to your child's life, rather than the only one solely responsible for its outcome.
2. Provide opportunities as often as you can that complement their abilities and passions, and try to guide them toward using their talents to make the world a better place. But don't be surprised when they don't want the same things you want or don't do things the way you would, because they don't and they won't.
3. No matter what, love them through it all, and make sure they know it.

Simple, apparently easy-to-follow guidelines like these are great fodder for how-to parenting books, which this clearly is not. So while I believe in these steps in theory, the reality of what it means to have two human beings depending on me for so much scares the hell out of me. I'm going to screw them up; I'm going to compare them; I'm going to shower them with affection sometimes when they do well and reflexively withhold it when they underperform.

Thank God that the human psyche and spirit are resilient and adaptable. If they weren't, it just wouldn't be fair for a neurotic guy like me, who hardly has his own shit together, to dare to be a parent. It sounds fatalistic, but part of my goal in all this is simply not to turn this blessing of new life we're offering to our children into a curse that keeps getting passed on down the line.

Amy and I have said, only half-joking, for years that the reason our marriage works is because we have so many great examples in our family history of what not to do. There's some twisted logic in looking back at your parents' failed marriages and doing the opposite. But parenting is a different ball of wax. You'll screw up, guaranteed, and more than once. But unless you're a complete tool, you never walk away from your kids. It can be a lifelong gift or a lifelong sentence, depending on how you play it.

CHAPTER 5

violent creation

Mattias: *I made a wish.*

Christian: *For what?*

Mattias: *For chicks.*

—Mattias, 3 years, 6 months

We debated about when to share the news of the new arrival with Mattias, partly because he has absolutely no filter for discretion but also because we weren't really sure how he would take it. He's made noise for some time about wanting a brother or sister, but he also talks about wanting a monkey, a violin, and a pair of sneakers that make him float in the air. You could occupy an entire zip code just with Mattias's wish list, so just because he says he's into being a big bro doesn't mean he really is ready.

We figured the best place to tell him was at his favorite restaurant: Souper Salad. How weird is that? How many four-year-olds do you know that get excited about eating a tray full of beets, cucumbers, peas, and carrots? I told you he wasn't normal. Anyway, we sat down to eat, and he was pretty wound up since we had told him earlier we had a surprise to share with him. He probably thought we got him a new Frisbee or something.

I leaned over and whispered to him that mommy had a baby in her tummy, and that he was going to be a big brother. He looked at me, eyes bulging, mouth hanging open, as if I'd punched him in the gut, and I anxiously waited for his brain to catch up to the information.

"Woo hoo!" he yelled, scaring a few nearby customers as he pumped his fists in the air. "Woo hoo!"

Whew. That wasn't so bad.

"I'm going to tell everyone that mommy has a baby in her tummy," he said, bouncing up and down in the booth, knocking a few carrots onto the floor. That, in a nutshell, is pretty much why we didn't tell him right away.

"You bet," I said, "go for it."

"Excuse me," he said to the waitress walking by, "my mom has a baby in there," pointing to her midsection, "and I'm going to be its brother."

"Wow, really?" said the young woman. "Congratulations."

"Yeah," he beamed, "and it's gonna come right out of her vagina."

I thought she was going to faint and fall face-first into his tuna skroodle. I mean the kid was right; if we're lucky, at least, the kid will be vagina-bound in about seven-plus months. I'm also proud of him for using proper terminology without shame, but remember the little thing I mentioned about no filter for discretion? That's what I'm talking about.

The whole exchange reminded me of Adam Sandler talking about the arrival of his second kid. "Don't worry," he said to his first kid, "Mommy's not really a bad kind of sick. She just has a creature growing inside of her that makes her throw up, then swell up really big. Then it'll come shooting out of her vagina, and it'll take half of your toys."

Don't get me wrong; I like me a vagina as much as the next guy, but right now, it's a source of no small amount of distress for me. After all, I was present at the birth of my first son, which, although it was an amazing miracle, was also pretty gross. It's not often that I see so much piss and blood at one time, and this was before the birth even took place. Watching things come out of the place that's supposed to be the ultimate object of desire for you is enough to put a guy off vaginas for a while. This was fine with Amy, by the way, as she had no interest at that time in my level of attraction to her goodies. But beware, guys, if you do the right thing and stand by your wife's side in the birthing room, you'll never look at her stuff quite the same way again.

As if that wasn't enough, the cesarian section showed me a whole other side of her that I'd never seen: the inside. It was surreal enough to see her liver, stomach, and intestines, and to watch the doctors push them around as they dug for the baby, but it totally weirded me out to watch this over the screen while, on the other side of the screen, Amy was talking to me. That's just not right.

The docs actually pulled her uterus out of her body and set it on her stomach in order to make a clean incision. Then all of a sudden, there's this other body in the room that wasn't there, at least officially according to the census, a minute ago. Then faster than I can put the first tiny little diaper on his butt, they've sewed her back up and put all the parts back in the right place. Now I know they've had a lot more practice at surgery than I had at diaper changing at the time, but the competitive side kind of looks forward to a rematch if it comes down to a C-section again.

Believe me, though, that is not my first choice. Amy and I have both come to believe that, although the doctors convinced us that inducing on a certain date was in our best interests, I actually wonder if her birth wasn't planned around the obstetrician's trip to Bermuda. I have no hard evidence, of course, that shooting her full of pitocin and forcing her body into labor before it was naturally ready had anything to do with the complications she experienced, but we've heard from more than one professional since then that his upside-down position in the womb could have been rectified naturally, and that a vaginal birth would not have been out of the question if she had not been induced.

There's something else. I remember the birth, along with everything before and after, in head-splitting detail. Amy doesn't. She was so full of painkillers that she kind of just floated through the whole experience in a haze. Though she knows that delivering naturally if she's able will be painful, she's decided that being more present to this one-in-a-lifetime experience is worth the short-term pain.

Once your wife has given birth, guys had better watch out. There's pretty much nothing left in your arsenal that will make you look tough, intimidating, or manly. I once passed a kidney stone and fell unconscious on the floor of my apartment. Granted, the thing was trying to come through my pee hole, but compared to a baby head, it was nothing. I was screaming like a schoolgirl every time that thing moved a little down the pipeline. I actually called my mom, who lived about an hour away at the time, and she drove all the way down to take me to the hospital.

Compare that to our friend, Marlene, from Colorado Springs, who came down to our house to deliver at the hospital across the street from us. She and her friends took a walk around the park *while she was in labor*. Once the contractions got close enough together, she went back by the house, picked up her bag, walked over to the hospital, and made a little baby deposit. Two days later, they came by our house, baby in hand, as if they had been on a little vacation for the weekend. Had that been me, I'd have been hooked up to ventilators with a steady morphine drip going twenty-four hours a day for at least a week.

I'll admit that although I'm not really a fan of seeing all kinds of stuff that I'd rather just stayed in there come out of one of my favorite spots, I do realize this time around that I'm beginning to look at Amy differently, even before she's starting to show any outward signs of pregnancy. In general, I look at her as my wife, friend, and partner, but now I look at her as this sort of mysterious temple for new life, which is something I'll never completely understand no matter how hard I try. The very fact that the human body can incubate another human being and then introduce it to the world to live on its own is as much evidence of the miraculous as I ever need.

It also reminds me that life is messy stuff. We are born in blood and piss, and forced violently into a new reality that is shocking and infinite. We arrive amid screams of pain, cries of joy, and whispers of wonder. We go in a single moment from being amphibious creatures, swimming in the protection of another body, to gasping for air, disoriented and flailing. We get squeezed, slapped, rubbed down, wrapped up and handed around, snipped, poked and measured until we're declared as official members of the human family. It's a violent ritual; one that speaks to the chaotic, unpredictable, wild nature of creation itself.

I wouldn't miss it for the world, even if the whole damn experience makes me want to submerge myself in a big vat of sanitizer and sit the whole thing out.

CHAPTER 6

mess manifesto

(Calling from the kitchen, while Mattias was playing with a balloon in the living room)

Me: *Mattias, are you OK in there?*

Mattias: *Yeah, I'm just in here being good, but I think the balloon pooped.*

—Mattias, 3 years, 1 month

I mentioned earlier that I'm not a big fan of messiness, which doesn't exactly go well with kids. I don't think there's been a single ten-minute stretch when our house has been officially clean since Mattias was born.

If you've ever played the old video game from the eighties called *Root Beer Tapper*, cleaning up a house with kids in it is kind of like that. Basically, there are five long bars in the game, each with a bunch of demanding customers craving some tasty root beer. Your job is to keep going back and forth from bar to bar, tossing mugs down the line to keep them from getting all the way to the end. But as soon as you take care of everyone up and down the line, a bunch of new ones pop up and you start all over again. That's the whole damn game and, I dare say, it's a metaphor for my whole damn life.

I have several matchbox-car-shaped scars in the soles of my feet from where I've firmly planted all of my weight on one of those bad boys in the middle of the night. I have shirts I've actually thrown away instead of trying to clean them from all the baby excretions I've gotten on them. I've also noticed I've lost a hell of a lot more hair in the past four years, which I'm pretty sure has a direct relationship to parenting.

All of this really is just the tip of the mess iceberg, though. It's probably easiest to lay this out in chronological order, starting with Amy while she was pregnant. Fortunately, this time around she hasn't had any morning sickness so far. By the way, the whole idea of morning sickness is a total fallacy, since the vomit really has no sense of time and comes any time of day really, usually when you're in a car, at a dinner party, or sometimes right in the middle of church.

I know it's kind of lame for me to complain about my wife throwing up since she's the one who suffers from it, but I'm what you might call barf-averse. I have two big fears in my life: going deaf and throwing up.

Amy hasn't had any morning sickness so far. Part of this can be chalked up to the fact that every pregnancy is different, but I'd also like to think we've learned a few things. For example, women are like Irish Setters when it comes to their heightened sense of smell while pregnant. Part of my job is to act as the radar man, scanning the perimeter for potentially offending sources of odor and then steering her well clear of any gag-inducing situations. Yesterday, we walked halfway across the grocery store parking lot to avoid two employees smoking on a bench by the front of the store: a surefire formula for spewage. Also, we've figured out that whenever she starts feeling queasy is precisely when she needs to eat something. We keep a good supply of granola bars and such on hand since these waves of nausea come with little warning and escalate to DEFCON 5 full-tilt barfing if not addressed quickly.

I guess it's "like mother, like son" when it comes to gastric issues, because Mattias was a hardcore sprayer for his first two years. There was one particular evening—the only time when we've taken him to the emergency room—when he threw up six or seven times in a row. He had pretty well blanketed every horizontal surface in the house with a film of puke, and he wasn't showing any signs of slowing down. We took him to the hospital and, of course, he promptly ceased all barfing activity. So we spent a couple of hours in the middle of the night sitting in a waiting room, only to be dismissed as hyperworried parents and sent back home.

We were so relieved, though, that he seemed to be doing better that we forgot what was waiting for us at home. The smell of puke knocked me in the face two steps into the door and nearly sent me into a barfing episode of my own. It was everywhere: on the sofa, across the dining room table, on both beds, and all over the bathroom. By then, it was about three o'clock in the morning and the last thing I wanted to do was clean up. But the stench was so overpowering there was no way we could sleep through it. Also, the idea of waking up to a house layered in dried-up vomit was too depressing to imagine. So I got to work.

It turns out that the puke was only part of the source of the smell. While we were gone, our dog, Maggie, got into a stash of dirty diapers and shredded them all across the upper level of the house. Also, she got into a bunch of strawberries that had gone bad that were in the trash. She scarfed them down, and then realized firsthand why it was that we threw them out in the first place. Not one to be left out of the puke parade, she promptly threw up half-digested strawberries all over the Asian rug in the dining room. If you hadn't drawn this conclusion on your own, strawberries mixed with canine stomach acid does not readily come out of a natural hair rug.

Suffice it to say I was ready to put a match to the whole place and walk away.

We got it relatively clean by about five in the morning and crashed for a couple of hours before Mattias woke up again. By then, we realized that he had passed his little gift on to us, so we took turns retching into a bucket for the next two days. I don't remember much about how we took care of Mattias during that time, but I'm pretty sure it had something to do with tossing him a giant box of Cheerios and sticking one Baby Einstein video into the DVD player after another.

Then there's the event that will forever be known as "The Pizza Mouse Incident" in our family. You know the place I'm talking about. Who ever thought it would be a good idea to have a rodent as a mascot for a restaurant anyway? What I ever saw in that godforsaken pit of pizza and evil, I may never know, but Mattias, just a toddler at the time, was pretty sure he had found Valhalla. He ran from place to place, eyes bigger than saucers, grabbing, throwing, and shrieking every few seconds. The fact that he had so much fun almost made it worth it, but if you've never been to a "pizza-and-carnival-games-for-kids" restaurant, you can't know the overstimulation hangover you're left with when you finally escape its grasp. My head was throbbing and Mattias was so spent he crashed in the back seat before we got to the highway. But Mattias sleeping in the car is a lot like sitting in the eye of a giant storm; you know the poop is coming and when it hits, it's going to get ugly.

This was an exceptionally volatile incident. As soon as the seatbelt clicked off in the driveway, you could see the fire well up in his eyes. I mean he was pissed. He started screaming so loud halfway to the door that I was worried someone might call us in for child abuse. My only crime, of course, was succumbing to the kitschy, hypnotic allure of a pizza joint on crack. Incidentally, we have never been back there again, and if I have any say about it, I'll never drop another dime in that hellhole. It's almost like we're asking for it going there in the first place. *Hey, come on in. We'll give you a subpar pizza to gnaw on while your kids get accosted by gigantic robotic mice and spend all your money. It'll be great!*

Anyway, we got him inside and were trying to get him upstairs to his room so we could get him in a diaper and pajamas. By this time, his face was blood red and puffy from screaming, and he was sputtering and gagging with every new shriek. Since this wasn't deterring us from our mission, he employed "spaghetti arms," which any parent will be familiar with. Basically, he let his entire body go limp while we're trying to hoist him up the stairs, so that he slithered out between our fingers. By the time we got to the first landing on the stairs we decided to take a break while Amy sat with him to try to calm him down. I ran up and got his clothes and she started trying to pry the ones he had off his writhing body.

By the time I got back to the landing, she had finally gotten his pants off, and just as I leaned in to try to wrap the new diaper around him, he let the water cannon fly.

He peed everywhere: on the wall, on the carpet, and on himself. If you've not witnessed the force behind a boy's pee stream, it's a thing to behold. My guess is that, if I had the same amount of force when I peed now, given my size, I'd be able to pee from my porch and water the neighbor's hedges. So in an effort to minimize the damage, I did the only thing I could think of; I went straight for the source with the diaper, trying to catch the spray and cut it off. Just as I leaned in, though, he did a nice little forty-five degree twist and turned his ammunition on me.

I should mention that I happened to be talking to Amy at the time, trying to get her to hold him still. His new move and my open mouth, however, made for a nasty combination. And I'm not talking about a couple of drops in the corner of the mouth either. I mean he easily hit the uvula before I knew what was going on and turned the other way.

Much to my surprise, the taste of kid-pee was not as revolting as I expected. It was more the idea that my son had peed in my mouth that was the real shocker. Amy nearly fell down the stairs laughing, while Mattias continued to yowl and writhe on the carpet, and I wiped my face and looked for somewhere to spit in a panic.

My only consolation is that I'll have this story as ammunition to share with his prom date or the like, just when he's primed for some humiliating parental anecdotes.

Although these make for good stories, they hardly compare with the real messiness that tends to keep me up at night. Most of my stress revolves around "what if" scenarios, which I can cook up, one after another, all day long. I know there's no benefit in dwelling on these what-ifs, but I can't seem to help it. It's almost like my mind has decided that worrying preemptively helps prepare me for every possible outcome, as if the worst thing in the world is to be surprised. The world is messy, unpredictable, aggressive, and even sometimes violent, and there's only so much I can do about it. People die, and as much as we try to sanitize it in our culture, it's usually ugly. Even worse than mismatched socks or a pile of kid puke, if you can imagine.

A recent news story helped punctuate my worry and, unfortunately, helped to validate keeping up the habit to some degree. A famous singer who has had three kids of his own, followed by three adopted kids from China, was at home with his children when his older son pulled into the long driveway toward the house in his SUV. Apparently the parents were paying enough attention to witness what happened next, but were not close enough to stop it. The young man ran right over his little adopted sister and she died shortly thereafter in the care of her doctors.

The story reminded me of a recent event at a fast food restaurant where we came across one of our friends and his three kids on the sidewalk outside. Now I won't say the name of the place where we were, but let's just say kids love it, and it smells of rampant capitalist imperialism and chicken nuggets, oozing from every crevice. Mattias loves our friend's kids, so they went nuts, running back and forth along the walkway, inventing improvised games, and then abandoning them for something more interesting no sooner than they had started.

This certain restaurant has a certain trademark lure that they use to draw your kids into beating you down until you take them: the infamous toy that comes with the kids' meal. This time the meal came with a car, which Mattias and the smaller other boy were launching off the side of a garden wall. It didn't take long until the toy predictably careened off the sidewalk and into an empty parking space a few feet away. More intent on the toy than on considering the risk to his own life, the little guy ran out into the parking lot after the car, just as a giant Hummer-type vehicle whipped around the blind corner and into the spot.

Though I had my back turned to the whole thing, Amy was watching it happen, and had lunged past me, screaming at the boy and waving her arms maniacally at the driver. The next thing I know, she jumped in between the car and the kid, as if her five-foot-four-inch frame would act as much more than annoying speed bump on the way in. By the time I turned around, I instinctively lunged toward the whole group too since, after all, why not give him more to run over? I knew she was pregnant, though, and even knowing I'd probably do the same thing if she wasn't there's something about a pregnant wife that makes a guy more than happy to beat the crap out of anything that threatens her safety, including inanimate objects like giant SUVs, apparently.

Lucky for all of us, he stopped short of squishing any of us, and we retrieved said pregnant wife, boy, and errant toy before any were harmed. But the whole event, which took no more than two or three seconds, sent my "what if" alarms into full alert mode for the rest of the evening. It helped to emphasize my relative inability to protect anyone I love, regardless of how hard I try.

This doesn't even skim the surface of the volatility of Mother Nature; she can be a real bitch sometimes. Though I have lots of friends who have had perfectly healthy pregnancies and deliveries, it seems like for every good story there's a tragedy. Just ticking through a quick mental list, I can think of friends who have dealt with the trauma of multiple miscarriages, infertility, premature deliveries, stillborn babies, and birth defects. I know others who have had to learn to live with the emotional aftershocks of having an abortion or giving up a child for adoption. Now some of these consequences are matters of choice, but so much is beyond our ability to choose.

For a neurotic like me, it's nearly enough to make me stop trying.

So remember how I mentioned I save my worry? Add in the stockpiling gene I acquired, and I've recently recognized I have a tendency to actually hoard anxiety and never throw any of my worries away. There was a time where I had no problem leaving every little thing where it fell, but my project now is to try my best to get rid of a few of my piles of worry. I'm honest enough with myself to recognize that I'll never go cold turkey, but I do believe it's worthwhile to limit the amount of time and energy I give worrying in my life. The metaphysical questions I'll never be able to answer definitely have to go on the junk pile, along with the things that give me ulcers, like worrying about what other people think of me. The "what if" pile is big and still growing, but that's the one I'm adding to the most these days.

As for the new baby, it's going to be what it's going to be. We can only do so much to increase the chances of a smooth pregnancy, an incident-free delivery, and a healthy fetus, but no contingency plans or stockpiles of worry stowed in the emotional corners of my brain are going to change the rest of it. And what if something weird happens? If the kid looks like a raisin, or has two heads, or worse, has a voice like Fran Drescher, am I going to love it any less? Of course not.

So at least for today, in preparation for the newest member of our family, my message to myself is to focus on the incredible opportunity to expand my ever-growing understanding of what love is, all the while recognizing that, in loving anything at all, you may get broadsided by an emotional Humvee.

Are we picking up what you're dropping here, God? If so, thanks a lot.

CHAPTER 7

vomit, bunnies, and "it"

If I go to the doctor, I'll say "Doctor, I don't feel so good. Oweeee."

—Mattias, 2 years, 8 months

Let the puking begin.

It wasn't me, in case you were worried, and technically it wasn't my wife either, actually. Some time around midnight last night I heard something akin to a potbellied pig being strangled within an inch of its life, but it turned out it was only my wife, dry heaving over the trash can next to me.

I got the telltale prickly things I get on my neck when someone so much as mentions barfing, but I did my husbandly duty and rubbed her back as she negotiated what was staying in and what was going out her gastric system. Turns out it all opted to stay, but not for lack of effort.

Though what came out of my mouth was, "Is there anything I can do for you, honey?" what was actually going through my mind was, "Why in the hell are you throwing up into a wicker trash can? Don't you know how incredibly gross that will be to clean up?"

As I said, it was a false alarm, and as pathetic as it may sound, I was pretty proud of myself for not either running out of the room or offering up a sympathy puke of my own. I felt a gurgle or two whenever she hit her highest, most resonant wretch noises, but I toughed it up and kept it all down.

Am I a swell husband or what?

You know the feeling, though, when you're so nauseous that you're about to hurl, but you just don't quite get there? That's more or less been Amy's reality for about the last ten days. By now with Mattias, she kept a baggie handy wherever she went in case one snuck up on her, but things have been tamer so far.

I say they've been tamer, but actually, a constant state of queasiness is more debilitating than just wailing on the toilet bowl for a few minutes and getting it over with. Oh, and it especially sucks when it happens during your first vacation together for a year and a half. I know, call me a jerk for thinking about my time off while she's laid up on the couch, feeling like crap, but I can't help it. It's not like I don't feel bad for her, but after a few days, the sympathy turns to fatigue, and you start thinking about how great it would be for you if this person you're caring for would just get better.

For anyone who's been around a pregnant woman during the first twelve weeks, there's pretty much a constant pendulum swing, back and forth between wanting to hurl and wanting to sleep. It does get better, which I'm glad I can still remember, at least by the second trimester, but she's hardly showing at all, so this cycle is pretty much the only evidence we have of the coming kid. Not much of a souvenir, I've gotta tell you.

So I've done my best to pick up the slack. I've taken on the dish washing and the laundry, and I've taken care of what little cooking we've done, since her weak stomach is hard to predict enough to plan a menu. I've been as patient as a self-centered male can be anyway, and she has definitely shown her appreciation. But here's the thing: we put off our annual vacation last year because of a lack of funds, so finally six months later, we got this sweet condo in Pagosa Springs, about three hours from our house, all to ourselves. And I'm happy for the baby coming and all, but this vacation was planned first.

Our favorite things to do when in Pagosa are to chill in the hot springs for hours every day, take some naps, have a couple of drinks on the porch at sunset, go out to eat, and maybe hit the springs again before bedtime. The thing is, she was not up for eating out, since she wasn't sure what she could keep down, and she's not had a drink since she found out she was pregnant. Strikes one and two. I figured we could at least put in some extra hang time at the springs, but the baby went and fracked that all up too. Turns out you're not supposed to let your body temperature go above a hundred degrees or so while pregnant, so we were relegated to the couple of lukewarm kiddie tubs instead of doing the ones we usually frequent.

As far as naps go, Amy was a champ. I don't think I've seen a human being not in a permanent alpha state who could sleep so much in a single day, then get up, brush her teeth, and head for bed. Practically speaking, I'm grateful that she had the down time when her body needed it, and that Mattias was staying with his aunt, uncle, and grandparents in New Mexico, keeping me from being otherwise overwhelmed. But do you remember back a few chapters when I said one of my concerns was that another kid would somehow get between us and our relationship? Well this bugger's no bigger than an olive and it's already a master nookie blocker, not to mention a class-A vacation-messer-upper.

This probably qualifies as another big worry of mine about having another baby. Not only do they not sleep when they're supposed to sleep and cry about pretty much everything, their digestive systems are possibly the most inscrutable mystery I've ever known. I had never seen so much puke in my life until I had a son. If there's anything that weirds me out the most about kids, it's puke, and not just that they barf a lot, but that they rarely give you any warning at all. Their eyes may bulge or glass over a bit, but more often than not, you'll get a spew-blanket in a matter of seconds, most likely right after you've put on a freshly ironed button-up shirt that's precisely the opposite color of the vomit.

If they had a vomit warning light or some other sort of early detection system, I'd be a much happier person. It would be especially great if the warning system gave me enough time to hand off the little guy to my wife, who doesn't seem to mind being barfed on. I, on the other hand, am much more likely to return the favor when covered with curdled milk. I'm funny that way.

But there are bigger problems. While we were in Pagosa, Mattias had his own adventures while playing with his favorite cousins, Miko and Michaela, down on his grandparents' fifteen-acre ranch in New Mexico. It's an amazing spot; beginning just feet off the Rio Grande river and extending up the side of a mesa across the small two-lane asphalt road. They have hundreds of apple trees in their orchard, along with horses, a donkey, some chickens, and more dogs than humans most of the time.

Amy's brother, Matt, and his family live across the road in a nice place they set up next to where the horses graze. They have a couple of dogs of their own, which are a curious pair. One is a Jack Russell named Che, after the revolutionary Che Guevara, although a Latin American radical is about the last thing you think of when you look at this thing. He's so lazy, he makes the pillows he's lying on look dynamic. Then there's Marley, a big mutt of about seventy-five pounds, who had a heart of gold until he suffered an attack from some of the local wildlife one night, followed by getting hit by a car a few months later. It's a wonder any dogs survive in this area, really, as reckless as the local drivers are and as proprietary as the coyotes and mountain lions are about their space. Little Che has probably only survived because he's too flabby and would hardly be big enough to serve as an appetizer.

Mattias has been warned not to mess with Marley too much since his accidents, as he's become pretty antisocial ever since. Miko has a scar over his right eye as a reminder of just that. But as long as you leave him be, Marley is generally content to lounge under the apple trees while life unfolds around him.

The farm is heaven for any kid, but according to the two cousins, Mattias just walked by and said "hello" to Marley, and the next thing you know, the dog had him pinned down and was gnawing at his face. By this time, of course, his cries of shock and panic had gotten everyone's attention and they came running, but Marley had no intentions of backing off. Little Miko, all of ten years old, grabbed a nearby chair and hurled it at Marley, who was too deep into "Cujo" mode even to notice.

By the time they pulled Marley off, Mattias was a basket case and was bleeding from several places on his chest and head. After cleaning him up and calming him down, the injuries weren't as serious as they could have been, but he did end up with a trip to the doctor, where he got his ear stitched and a tetanus shot.

"I don't like that dog one bit," pouted Mattias. "Send him to Australia." We had told Mattias that Australia was about as far away as you could get and still be on the planet, so he decided this was a good plan.

Matt, however, decided that Australia might not be far enough away. "I love that dog," he said solemnly over the phone, "but I love my nephew more." Matt loaded Marley up in the car, along with his pistol and a shovel, and drove out to some open property controlled by the Bureau of Land Management.

Talk about a scene straight out of *Old Yeller*. Though I think he did the right thing putting the dog down, I don't know if I could have done the same thing. But Matt's a do-it-yourself kind of guy, and his feeling was that it's his dog, so it's his responsibility. Why hand over a job to a vet that should be handled by the owner. It's strange to think of something so sad and violent as an act of love, but it really was just that.

If parenthood teaches you anything, it's that life isn't about you anymore. We all carry that little child around inside ourselves still; you know, the one that still hollers, "Hey, what about me?" when your kid gets the biggest piece of cake, or your vacation plans change, or any countless number of other things that make you realize you're not really as important and special as you'd like to be. First and foremost, from now until death, you are a parent. You're a caretaker, provider, nurturer, teacher, guide, occasional inspirer, and reluctant judge. More than fulfilling the dreams for your own world, you lay yourself down for the dreams of others that will come after you, and perhaps for the first time, you begin to think about what the world will be like after you're no longer a part of it.

There's something suddenly more important than life itself, though ironically it is life itself, just not as you pictured it. You feel the pain in others more than you sense your own pain, and all you wish for is to take it on so they don't have to bear it. There's more than a small amount of insanity in signing on to parenthood. The pay sucks, for one, although the benefits are something else.

We met Amy's mom, Suzie, at the little diner in Fort Garland, Colorado, where Amy and I stopped only a few minutes after we got engaged more than nine years ago. Though little has changed about the little greasy spoon on the rim of the San Luis Valley, there were two very important additions to my life waiting inside to see us. When that scratched up little face turned around and met eyes with mine, nothing else mattered. Those arms clung around my neck with all the love, faith, and trust in the world, even though I hadn't been there for him when he got mangled. In fact, he was busting at the seams to show off his single blue stitch, poking out from the back of his ear. He beamed as he lifted his Denver Broncos jersey to his chin, revealing the battle scars he bore on his chest.

What had been for me a yoke of guilt for the past three days was already an exciting anecdote for him. He reveled in recounting how he didn't even cry when the thread was inserted in his ear, and that even though the tetanus shot was less than pleasant, he was a trooper for that too. I was proud of my little guy, and after seeing him all in one piece, I allowed myself to lay the yoke down, at least until after lunch.

Not one to pass up a chance for a nap, Amy konked out on the way over La Vita Pass on the way back to Pueblo. As Mattias perused his book on Spanish words for body parts in the back seat, I breathed a little sigh of relief and whispered a couple of thankful words to myself, glad to have my family all back together again and headed home, where we belong.

Next week is Amy's first sonogram, which is an exciting but emotionally loaded event. First off, you should see this thing they stick up in there to take pictures of your baby. You'd think, with the invention of all the fiber optic cameras and microspy devices, they could come up with something that doesn't give every husband an inferiority complex. Then there's the fact that someone you've never met before is going places with this phallic device where only you normally go.

You've probably noticed that, up to this point, there's not much warm and fuzzy stuff about this new baby. That's because, for guys, it's a total abstraction until you have more physical proof. We men are fairly literal creatures when it comes down to it, and some bigger boobs, though wonderful, do not give us The emotional connection a woman has to some other living being, growing inside her womb.

That's why the sonogram is such a big deal. It's not even that you suddenly look at this little blob and see yourself in it. It actually looks more like a half-melted salamander than a human at eight weeks or so. We actually like to joke that "it has your eye," or "it has my tail," but there's no doubt it's a real live thing in there, even if it's not very person-like yet.

It's kind of weird to call your own baby "It," but at this point, and for at least another month and a half, we won't know the sex. I've proposed a gender-neutral name like Farfel or Mutt until we know better, but Amy's not a fan of my proposal. So for now, it's an "It."

One thing about the sonogram that's so emotionally loaded is that that level of abstraction I've enjoyed up to now begins to dissolve. It's not just an idea or a plan for our future anymore; it's a sort-of human. Part lizard and part tadpole, but definitely part human too.

There's a part of me that admittedly is resistant to loving It. After all, loving in itself is a vulnerable act, and who wants to be so vulnerable to something so fragile and dependent itself? There's this little part of me that says *wait, let's see how this plays out, and if things go well, I'll love It.* But that's not the deal. For some reason I can't help it. Ideally, the love would displace the neuroticism and resentment about the changes that are coming, but instead they kind of comingle into a big, messy lump of complicated emotions. Is it possible to love something while also fearing it and holding a grudge because it simply exists?

Apparently so.

One night recently Amy started having some cramps in bed. As if this wasn't enough to get me a little worried, the look on her face put me over the top. All we could do was lie there and wait. I reached over and put my hand on her lower abdomen, and said a little silent prayer. *God, take care of my family* was all I could come up with. Thankfully the pains subsided after a while and she was able to sleep. But it was yet another reminder of the foolishness of loving someone. It's not logical. It doesn't make sense. But it's in our nature.

It's tapping into that love part of our nature that makes life both worth living and so completely certain to fall apart.

CHAPTER 8

daddy day conspiracy

Frankenstein has just a little bit of hair, just like you, daddy.

—Mattias, 2 years, 11 months

What jackass invented Fathers' Day?

We were headed to church an hour-plus before anyone else arrived to make sure everything was in order, and the first volunteer showed up about half an hour later and promptly wished me a happy Fathers' Day.

"It's Fathers' Day?" Mattias said looking up from the drums he was playing with on the floor.

"Sure is," I said, waiting for my big hug.

"Huh," he shrugged, and wandered off to something else more interesting.

On Mothers' Day, we give all the women at church flowers to honor their dedication. Father's Day, however, made about as much of a collective impression as a fart in a fan factory. Come to think of it, I don't even think we mentioned it.

Afterward, we had two more commitments that would keep us busy the rest of the day, and I began to realize there was likely no surprise card, gift, or special dinner to come. Hell, I would have even settled for a crappy piece of macaroni art or something, but instead we just kept up our streak, several weeks running, of doing stuff for other people.

I finally reached my peak of self-pity while driving down the road to our first stop when I stubbornly announced I had no intention of going. Amy was sick after we had spent a grueling week wrangling more than seventy kids at a summer camp and we were both wiped out. Amy suggested she might just take a nap in the back room while I watched Mattias at the lunch where we were headed, and that's the very moment when something small but very hot snapped somewhere around the base of my skull.

"No," I said.

"What?"

"Screw it. I'm not going," I insisted. "I don't have to and I'm not going to." I felt like I was about five years old saying it, but it's how I felt and I was simply at my limit.

"But we have to go," she said. "I already told everyone we'd be there."

"Then you can go." I was really pouring on the childishness, but why stop now? By the time she picked up her phone to call and cancel, I felt kind of like a douche, but it wasn't like I could take it back now. Besides, I was getting my way, right?

"Fine," she said, dialing the phone, "we can go wherever you want."

"If you're too tired," I said, trying after the fact to soften the edges of my attitude, "we can just go home. I don't want you to go somewhere just because you feel like you have to." This was a lie, but if she was going to spend the whole afternoon being pissed off at me, I wanted her to feel at least a little bit guilty about it.

"No," she sighed, "it's Fathers' Day, and we didn't get to do anything for you since we've been gone, so we can do this at least."

Fair enough. I'll take it. I picked a restaurant, which Mattias promptly tried to shoot down.

"I don't want to go there," he whined. "Why do we have to go there?"

"Because it's Fathers' Day," I snapped, "and because we didn't plan anything else, and because I'm the dad and we're going to do what I want for a change!" The car was unusually quiet on the way to eat after that, which would have been nice had it not been because everyone else was afraid of tipping me over the edge into a mass killing spree.

After I filled my stomach and crashed on the couch for a much-needed rest, I started to gain some perspective about my outburst and what was behind it. Most obviously, I'm still working through the issues between me and my dad. I'd love to say I'm past it, but honestly, how do you get past not speaking with a parent? And although most days being a dad myself is great, the negatives are only magnified by a holiday focusing on the particular parent in question that's not around.

On top of that, it inevitably raises any lingering doubts I have about my own parenting ability. After all, who else influenced my idea of what a dad is supposed to be like more than my own father? And it's not that my entire childhood experience was negative, but let's just say the third act isn't playing out exactly as I had expected. Considering, also, the trends that preceded me on his side of the family, the odds of me actually doing my job well as a dad are not good.

The fact that I practically had to lie on the ground and throw a fit to go out to eat on Fathers' Day also points to how busy our lives already are. To be fair, we did take a vacation a couple of weeks ago for the first time in about eighteen months, but as I already mentioned, Amy was laid up with baby-itis most of the time. Once we got back, we were not only a week behind from being gone, but we had to plan ahead for the week we'd miss after that since we'd be at the youth camp. So that whole week in the middle was more or less insane. Not only was I buried under a huge project for work, but Amy was still kind of puny from the bambino, so I was also pulling overtime on kid and housekeeping duty.

The good news about the youth camp is that it was a great experience, apparently for all involved. The bad news is that it was, like most things we get involved with, a lot of work. Amy had to go up to the camp early since she was the director, which left me to handle church by myself before driving straight up to the forest after services. And of course, about twelve hours after we got home from camp, church hit again, which also happened to be on Fathers' Day. As a bonus, Amy was sick from some crap a snotty kid shared with her or something, so again, I have been doing a little extra to keep things from coming unraveled.

It's obviously not Amy's fault that she's had no time or energy to plan anything for Fathers' Day, but the selfish little voice in my head tells me that I definitely deserve something. How can I just let this day dedicated to swell guys like me go by without some official stamp of approval to validate my fatherly efforts? Also, how are we ever going to have time to do even a half-assed job raising another kid if we can't even find the energy or time to celebrate a lame holiday invented by a greeting card company?

Honestly, where have our priorities gone?

I know, it's not really that big of a deal because I hardly ever wear ties and macaroni art really is a tragic waste of good food. However, this contrived, superficial blip on the calendar somehow represents so much more. It gets bogged down in all of my old family baggage, my neuroses about being a good dad, my frustrations about making time for my marriage, my freak-outs about money, and a million other things.

On a good day, I can either keep all of this from boiling over in my best maintenance mode, or I can at least find enough emotional reserves to suppress the feelings that seep to the surface, to be dealt with later. At the risk of beating an already overused cliché more to death, Fathers' Day this year just happened to be my perfect emotional storm.

Then I thought back to a friend of mine recently. His name is Mark and he has Tourette's syndrome, though as he points out, it's not the cool kind where you shout obscenities at highly inappropriate moments. He does, however, struggle with a significant stutter and a number of quirky physical tics. Underneath all of that is an incredibly sharp-witted, sensitive, and funny guy, though for some it's hard to get past the surface stuff. He recently landed a teaching gig with kids who have special needs, but his career aspirations have not historically lived up to his potential, in large part because of his condition.

He talked candidly to a rather large group of us about his syndrome, and some of the emotional and social fallout that has accompanied it. Even recently, he struggled with a spell of depression, waking up more down every day than he had been the day before. But then one day, he came to the realization that, if he indeed had less hope today than he had yesterday, then that means he had at least a little bit of hope the day before. In becoming aware of this, he actually carried that tiny bit of hope over into the present day, nurturing it into something a little bit more substantive. A few days later, some momentum had built up around this and he was more or less out of his depression strictly based on an act of personal will. He could justifiably give up because he had less than he wanted, but instead he focused on what he had, however little it seemed to be.

Now if that doesn't make you feel like a tool for feeling sorry for yourself, nothing will.

I started to think about all the people, just in my immediate circle of friends and acquaintances, who either have never known their fathers at all or whose dads died prematurely. It's not that I feel better knowing there are people who are worse off than I am, but somehow that bit of perspective caused me to reflect on the best times I could remember with my dad.

Like the time when I was so sick on Halloween that I couldn't go trick-or-treating, so he brought an enormous bag of candy home from the store and buried me in it while I lay in my bed.

Or when he gave me a special "Hustle Award" one year when I worked my ass off in middle school soccer, even though I still sucked.

Or the year when my mom was in the hospital on her birthday, and even though I was about seven years old and no one under the age of twelve was allowed on her floor, he smuggled me in to wish her a happy birthday.

There are tons more that come to mind the longer I think about them, like how he bought me a set of drums on his fortieth birthday, and how he was the only one who flew halfway across the country to see me receive my master's degree. He taught me how to use tools, he helped me rebuild my '66 Mustang, and he taught me every disgusting joke I knew before the age of fifteen. We hiked into the Colorado Mountains together, where I learned more about what I could do as a man than I expected, and we used to cut sprigs of mistletoe from neighborhood trees at the holidays when I was little so I could sell them for gift money.

So yeah, he's not around, and no, he hasn't responded to any of my e-mails or cards in a couple of years. Sure, he's said and done things to distance himself from me and most of the other people I care about, but he's my dad, and he's the only one I have, like it or not. Though I definitely have less hope for the future of our relationship today than I did a couple of years ago, I guess the very fact that I have less hope at all suggests there was hope to lose, which, in a weird way, is something to celebrate.

Whether that's enough to take from here forward and reinvent fatherhood as I want it to be is, I suppose, up to me.

CHAPTER 9

the cha-cha

Hair on naked parts is great!

—Mattias, 3 years, 2 months

Amy looked her rapidly mutating body up and down in the full-length mirror. "There's stuff coming out of my boobs," she sighed.

"Do you know how much of a turn-on that is?" I said.

"Yeah, I don't really care."

I pretty much expected that kind of reaction, but you simply can't let that sort of comment go by without a response, now can you?

You also can't very well write a book about pregnancy and childbirth and not talk about sex. But having a kid around the house, we've learned to discuss such things in a sort of code; being fans of *Dancing with the Stars* (don't judge me—I know you watch it too), we went with dance metaphors. I'm fine with talking birds and bees with Mattias, but I think the image of his parents copulating might sear a permanent hole in his psyche at his age. Well, I have news for you, son, should you be reading this some day in the future: we parents don't check our genitals at the gate when we start raising kids; we hang on to them with every intention of putting them to use, thank you very much.

But to provide at least some veneer of protection for his mental health, let's just say we love to "cha-cha."

Most guys figure that you might as well hang up your dancing shoes for nine months after you slip one past the goalie, as there will be no cha-chas going on under your roof for many moons. Pregnancy, however, has about the same effect on the female sex drive as global warming seems to have on the climate: it certainly changes things, but exactly how it will change is nearly impossible to predict.

The last time I suggested a little cha-cha, I got a look like I had just blown a fart under the covers. So I resolved from then on to keep my cha-cha desires to myself. That worked well enough until one morning Amy announced that she had trouble sleeping during the previous night.

"I really wanted to cha-cha all of a sudden," she said, "but I didn't know if I should wake you up or not." Now there was a time when I would have no problem answering this question, considering that opportunities to sleep are nearly infinite, while cha-cha hour is a much more limited engagement. However, at thirty-six, the idea of doing the cha-cha instead of sleeping caused me more than a moment of pause.

"Let me get back to you," I said. "I have to think about it."

"OK."

"You don't still want to cha-cha, do you?"

"Not really, no."

"Dammit. Didn't think so."

The next day, Amy went up to take a nap while I was working, when I suddenly heard a call to cha-cha coming from upstairs. Given a choice between work and cha-cha, the decision is much easier.

The problem is that doing the cha-cha is, well, sort of like dancing. If you don't cha-cha for a while, it may take a while to get back in the groove. But if your partner is already set to cha-cha whether you are or not, you may be left in the dust.

Plus, have you ever tried to dance with someone else always trying to cut in? The cha-cha is a particularly private dance, and to have the yet-to-be-named "It" hogging the dance floor is a little bit distracting. Some guys actually find pregnant women to be a turn-off altogether, which is not a problem for me. In fact, like I mentioned before, it's about as close as a guy can come to cheating and still keep his marriage intact. You basically go to bed with a new woman every night, although you're never sure if that woman will want to jump your bones, tie your junk in a knot, or just throw up in a trash can.

So the trick is how to stay on high cha-cha alert in case the call comes unexpectedly without imploding in a puddle of sexual frustration. It's not as easy as you might think either, given that even the basic routines you may generally use to prepare for a cha-cha may be off the table.

For example, Amy and I finally planned an evening out alone last night. It was the first time since she was laid up a few weeks ago in Pagosa that we had time to ourselves, and the only time in about a month or more when she felt well enough to go out when we did have the opportunity. Amy's aunt offered to take Mattias for the evening, and we headed out to one of our favorite local pubs for dinner. Everything was going well until she got that curious look on her face, sort of like a puffer fish about ready to fend off a predator.

"You feeling OK?" I asked, more concerned at the time about losing a free night out than anything. Amy just offered a puny smile, trying to keep her game face on.

"'I'll be all right," she said. "Just need to take it easy." OK, so the roller derby and the feats of strength I had planned for the night were a no-go. I could handle that. We decided to go over to a coffee shop to hang out on the patio and chat.

That's when the gas started to hit.

That's when I knew our night on the town was toast.

By the time I retrieved Mattias from the sitter, put him to bed, and came down to join her on the couch, I knew better than to even mention the word "cha-cha." Had I done so, I'm pretty sure I'd have been told to go cha-cha myself for the indefinite future.

Sexuality is one of the things that bring out both the best and worst in the complexity of human nature. While most other creatures do their thing simply to keep the production line going, we have the potential to get so much more out of it. Rather than doing little more than offering the equivalent relief of a sneeze below the belt, we fold in a good deal of our identities, both as individuals and as couples, with our sexuality. Hell, we even take our sexual impulses to the legislature, making what we do with our naughty bits a matter of national public interest. We have—at least many of us do at one time or another—a substantial emotional investment in the person with whom we engage sexually, and whereas a duck or a cat might have parental responsibilities for a few days or months, parenthood changes our lives forever.

There's also plenty of opportunity for sex to be misappropriated. From children becoming victims of older sexual predators to the way we treat people of different sexual orientations, the victims of sexuality seem at times to number as many as those who benefit from it. There's sexual addiction, made even more prevalent with the internet, along with the popularly acceptable objectification of young women. Relationships have been made and broken over sexual matters, and, far too often, children are being born to other children, hardly at an emotional, financial, or spiritual place in their lives to give their progeny the kind of life they deserve.

Given all of this, I guess that the frustration of our sexual clocks being a bit out of sync doesn't seem like such a big deal. There is some irony, though, in a previous sexual act having such profound repercussions on subsequent acts, or nonacts, as it were. As much as I like irony, right now, I'm thinking it pretty much sucks.

But despite the frustrations and mild inconveniences, the best part has to be bearing witness to this relatively slow but incomprehensible development process. Every single day, Amy becomes a little bit more of something else—or someone else—giving entirely of herself to this other life that is so completely dependent on her that it simply can't survive without her.

There is no bond more incredibly powerful than that of a mother and an unborn child. Sure, it may hamper my afternoon delights for a while, but I suppose getting the chance to see life emerge, right before my eyes, is a miracle worth waiting for.

Right now, this little miracle is giving me a horrible case of blue balls.

CHAPTER 10

talking death

*Oh God, please don't be invisible. I don't know how to
do this. Please don't let all the bees sting me. I don't want
to die. Please don't let everybody die. Please don't let me
be a big pile of ashes that the people put on their heads.
Please don't be invisible. I can't do this. I'll just die and
be with you. Please, God.*

—Mattias, 4 years, 5 months

I've noticed that Mattias has been more fearful in general lately, which concerns me. Part of it, I think, has to do simply with the fact that he's smart enough to think through possible scenarios. As I've observed with him a number of times before in the last two years, he's able to process a whole lot more intellectually than he can process emotionally. Eventually, his emotional wisdom should have plenty of opportunity to catch up, but for a four-year-old, any gap in development is more pronounced.

Two years ago, when he was only a year and a half old, Mattias was jumping from the side of the pool into my arms and going underwater. Last summer, he and his cousin spent most of every waking hour in their grandmothers' pool, diving to the bottom for toys and to do tricks. Now with floaties on both arms, a mask, and a snorkel, it's all I can to do get him off of the top step in the shallow end.

What the hell happened?

I think it has something to do with all the questions about death he's been asking lately. He asks about when he's going to die, when his mom and I will die, what happens to our bodies, and since we're spiritual folks, where our souls go. Is God waiting for us somewhere else? Why do we have to die? How long will we live, and when we die, will worms eat our brains?

Then we got down to the good stuff.

"Daddy," he asked, "if you and mommy die, do I have to go live somewhere else?" I explained, in as much of a matter-of-fact tone as I could muster, that he would live with me if mommy died, and with her if I died, but that it wasn't something he had to spend any energy worrying about. But he wanted to know what the plan was if we both got whacked at the same time. I told him he'd live with his grandparents in New Mexico, which only led him to wonder where he'd go if they died. This went on and on through the familial chain until there were few, if any, of us left. I couldn't help but picture the apocalyptic scene, with all the Piatts, Pumphreys, Robinsons, Brendles, and so on all laid out in coffins side-by-side, with my little guy looking worriedly on.

Not a pleasant scene, but what are you going to do when your kid brings it up? I felt like I owed him an answer, to a point, at least. By the time he had about a dozen and a half of us knocked off in his imagination, I told him that was about as far down the line as we'd planned, but that he was incredibly lucky since he had so many family members and friends who wouldn't hesitate to love him and take care of him in our absence.

Now Mattias's latest plan is not to have any more birthdays. He's decided that the cake, presents, and all the attention are heavily outweighed by the grim reaper leaning in over his shoulder. I admire his resolve to hold off the inevitable by ignoring cultural landmarks like birthdays, but I haven't had the heart to tell him he's still going to die someday, whether he ever puts on another pointy party hat or not.

It sucks, though, watching him struggle with the realities of life, which also include the eventual absence of all we now love and treasure, especially at such a young age. It seems like a bit of a cruel joke we've played on him, bringing him into a world we knew had such glaring flaws.

Here, kid. Have a nice life. Embrace it all and live like there's no tomorrow, because, someday, there will be no tomorrow. It might be today, and it might be a hundred years from now, and you'll never know until it's right on top of you. But don't let everything getting taken away from you stop you from foolishly throwing yourself into this fickle, fragile existence that someday will turn on you and convert you and all you love to compost. Muah, hah, haaaah!!!

We all suffer from a terminal condition called life. It's unavoidable, and in some ways, bringing another life into a world bound by the rules of death seems unfair. Imagine the doctor who delivered you standing over your first crib, shaking his head. "I'm afraid she's going to die," he says, "and it's not something she's going to be able to recover from, ever."

Bummer, right? That's kind of how I feel about it right now, getting all these questions about death from my four-year-old while waiting on the arrival of another little victim. I know, I'm being morbid and overly dark, but the only other option, at least for me, is not to deal with death at all, which is about the most brazen form of denial I can think of.

Unfortunately, it took me a long time to come to terms with death, as it wasn't something we dealt with very much in my house growing up. I remember breaking down at the dinner table while opening presents on my thirteenth birthday, effectively turning a celebration into a wake for my childhood. It also didn't help that, during my grade-school years, I had youth leaders in church who bluntly informed me that my dad would not be joining us in the big party in the sky when he kicked the bucket. Thanks for that one, folks.

There's a line from a song that's been one of my favorites for a number of years, performed by a band called Semisonic. They sing, *"Every new beginning comes from some other beginning's end."* The crappy part is that we have to end the old things sometimes before we can get started on the new ones. It's sort of like wanting a cookie we can't see inside of a jar, but not wanting to lay down the carrot we have in our hand to be able to reach in and see what we get. Who, after all, wants to let go of the certainty of the carrot for the possibility of a cookie?

It's ironic that we have to accept, as fully as we can, our own death to truly live, but that's part of the poetry of life. Life is a constant series of little, tiny births, and deaths; we die to life in the womb and are reborn into the world; we die to childhood and emerge as adults; we die to our fears and awaken to the hope and promise of a life unbound by that same fear. Life is still a gift, no matter how long it lasts. We can't assess the validity a life strictly based on tenure. Instead, we have the chance to celebrate each person's involvement in an ongoing, miraculous event, of which we are a startlingly small part.

Eventually, our cards will all be punched, and even the most "important" of us will be forgotten. It's really only a matter of time. For some, they will become no more than faces in a scrapbook within a few decades. For others, it may be hundreds of years before they become more historic myth than fact.

The point, it seems to me, is not to compete for the biggest imprint on the collective memory of history, but rather to live as fully as possible into one day only: today. There's a great moment in the movie *Kung Fu Panda* when the old, toothless turtle offers a bit of wisdom to his protégé, who is feeling like his life has not added up to what it should have.

"Yesterday is history," he says, "and tomorrow is a mystery. All we have is today, which is a precious gift. That's why it's called 'the present.'"

OK, I just threw up in my mouth a little after typing that, but cliché or not, I wish I'd thought of it first. Guess that's why I haven't gotten the call to write dialogue for any talking cartoon animals yet. Any day now though, I bet.

Meanwhile, I'll be here, the man I need to be at least for today, just living the dream.

CHAPTER 11

pain and suffering

Will the girls in the coconut bras kiss me, then smack me in the face?

—Mattias, 3 years, 5 months

When I first found out I was going to be a dad, I was relieved my first kid was a boy. First of all, I was more than a little concerned that a girl would dominate me like Shaq on a point guard and I'd have no chance of being a serious authority figure. Fortunately, I think I have enough practice under my belt to keep my game face on, even if the new baby is a girl and learns how to flash doe-eyed glances my way. I'll be a sucker, no doubt, but at least I have five years of training now.

The other thing I worry about is how I would ever let go of a little girl enough to let her live her own life. After all, having been a guy for pretty much my whole life, I know a good deal about how guys act, what they want, and what they try to do with girls, especially once they get boobs. As I said, boobs are awesome, but if I have a kid with boobs, any boys' hands who so much as brush against them, even by accident, should promptly wither up and fall off.

It's not that girls are inherently more emotionally vulnerable than boys, but there's this deep, dark part of being a dad that just makes me want to dismember any guy who glances at my baby girl. I don't even have a girl—at least not yet—but I know that part of me is in there somewhere. It is kind of strange that I don't have quite the same degree of protectiveness about Mattias, especially considering how sensitive he is, but the little voice in your head just tells us guys, for some reason, that he'll tough it out and what doesn't kill him will make him stronger. So by that logic, then, my job as his dad is to allow him to endure as much pain and suffering as he can stand, short of death, so he'll grow up to be a stronger man, right?

It sounds really stupid when you say it out loud, and I'm still not really sure where the healthy balance is between letting him learn from his own experience—pleasant or not—and protecting him from unnecessary hurt. God knows there's more than enough hurt in this world to go around.

There are all different kinds of pain, and I guess I react differently to each situation. For example, he came home and told me the other day about a boy in his class who made him cry because he told him he didn't want to be his friend. *Screw him*, I'm thinking to myself. *Move on, shake the dust off your feet, and don't give him any satisfaction for being a little jerk.*

But he needs more than that from me, so we talked about ways to handle this kid. After a couple of days, it turns out that they are best friends again, so I guess the coping tools worked this time. There are other times when Mattias's mouth has written checks his little four-year-old butt was not ready to cash and, in those cases, as long as the offended party has no weapons, I say my kid has a lesson to learn.

I've watched more than one bigger boy knock him down or even bloody his nose because of some smartass comment he made. So do I play Old-Testament God and let the judgment fall as it may, or do I go more New Testament and focus on responding to aggression with peace? And how, exactly, do you teach such an unnatural response to a little kid who's getting the snot beaten out of him? Part of me wants to jump in and thump his aggressor for him; the other part of me just wants to hug him and make all the bad stuff go away.

The sooner I figure out a decent answer, the better, because the older he gets, the higher the stakes will be.

This kind of concrete, physical pain actually is pretty easy for most guys to handle, especially with a son. The emotional pain is a little bit more complicated. Fortunately, he's still too young to have anything more than little flirtations with girls now and again, but the day will come soon when he'll fall hard, only to have his little kid-nuts stepped on by someone he cares about. But the pain is the same regardless. How do you prepare a kid for that kind of hurt?

The quote at the top of the chapter was from a trip to Hawaii we took a little bit more than a year ago. Mattias somehow got obsessed with the hula dancers who wear coconut bras. I guess he has some innate sense of the potential power of the weiner-tease. Once you let a girl get ahold of you—whether literally, hormonally, or emotionally—be ready for some yanking. He's going to get hurt by someone, and more than likely by a lot of someones. So to what degree is it my job to shelter him from possible pain or fear, and at what point is that protection doing more harm than good?

Clearly, I have no clue.

We were at the park the other day where they have these kiddie rides the children can ride for a quarter. It's always a favorite summer outing for Mattias, and we enjoy it too. He digs the train, the little motorized cars that perpetually go in a circle, and the rockets that spin in pretty much the same way. For the last two years, he's also enjoyed the roller coaster, which couldn't be more than fifty feet from beginning to end, and which maybe reaches six feet at its highest point. He's been riding it since he was two, but all of a sudden, he balked at the idea of riding, while his friend went ahead and did it on his own.

By the end of the night, he thought he could brave the coaster if I rode it with him, so I agreed. But as soon as we got to the front of the line, he pulled a Rain Man on me, wailing and screaming that there was no way in hell he was getting on that mechanized beast of death, in so many words at least. Needless to say, I was both frustrated by the fit and annoyed about having waited in line for nothing, but I also realized a third emotion I had not felt about him before: shame.

It actually embarrassed me that my kid was flailing on the sidewalk while little girls two years younger than he was toddled right on to the platform. I started to wonder what the other dads thought about me and about what kind of a boy I was raising. All of a sudden, his hang-ups about some stupid kiddie ride became a reflection on me as father.

I was talking to my mom about this, and she brought up that this episode, along with several of the fearful things I talked about in the previous chapter, had occurred after he was attacked by the dog in New Mexico. It also is not inconsequential that we're going back there next week for a visit and that he's been asking us daily about Marley's whereabouts. God forbid he'd return from his sabbatical in Australia to unleash more canine fury on my kid's face. I think he understands that Marley's no longer a threat, but I've tried to put myself in Mattias's shoes since then, imagining what it must have been like to have a dog twice your size pin you down and dine on your face. This, of course, was followed up by stitches and shots too, which are hardly a fitting reward for bravery either.

Of course he's scared. It's the closest to death he's ever come. He still has the scars on his face, and returning to the scene of the attack is probably a little bit terrifying. To top it all off, I wasn't there to rescue him when he was at his most vulnerable, so now, when he's working out his feelings about it all, I take it personally and worry about what everyone else thinks of my parenting. But as my dad used to say, you can worry in one hand, take a crap in the other, and see which one fills up first. I have no idea what this is supposed to mean, but I've always assumed it was his mellifluous way of telling me what all my worry amounted to.

It's not the end of the world that he got hurt. It's not the first—or hardly the last—time it will happen either. Though it is my job to help him avoid unnecessary, excessive pain, it's neither my job, nor even a realistic possibility, to expect to offer him a pain-free existence.

Right now, it's a delicate balance between patience as he sorts out his own place in the world and not letting him get too comfortable with his own fears. Pain, after all, is not the worst thing that can happen to him; living in constant fear of pain is a hell of a lot worse. So I can spend all my time and energy protecting him from pain, but if he still lives his life in the shadow of fear, I've failed him.

Meanwhile, as I'm still trying to figure this stuff out with number one, the sequel is on its way. Brilliant.

Still, I'm not too worried my little guy won't develop at least some of the Piatt fighting spirit. I'm generally a pretty understanding guy, but the other day when we finally had our first appointment with our doctor for the ultrasound, he sashayed into the room without so much as a "howdy do" and proceeded to plunge head first into the holy of holies. He didn't even have on a white lab coat, or a stethoscope handing around his neck, or anything. For all I knew he was some bored husband who wandered into the wrong room and decided to go exploring. And despite my immediate inclination to bash his head in, though, I held myself in check and played it cool. And I had to give the guy props for how good he was with the camera thingy.

Though we still won't know for a few more weeks whether the kid has an "innie" or an "outie" junk-wise, it's looking more like something quasi-human, and less like a turd with arm buds.

I couldn't help but go soft watching the little heart pound away on the monitor, putting everything it has into growing and making its way toward joining us in the world. Thinking ahead to January, even the very moment of birth is drenched in pain. You want to take the pain on yourself, or avoid it all together if you can, but without the pain there's no life. Fortunately, life is much more than just pain, but strangely life cannot be what it is without at least a little bit of suffering.

I guess the Buddhists got it right when they said "life is suffering." At first I thought this was a particularly depressing concept, but then I

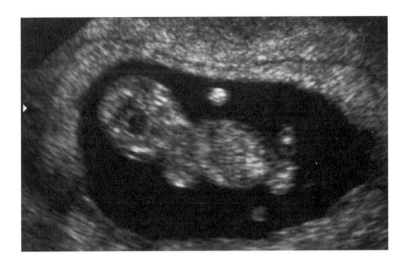

realized what they meant was that trying to avoid suffering is to avoid life. Embracing one's pain and growing from it helps life move forward.

I don't want to see my kids hurt, but I'd choose a little pain over having them miss out on the only chance they have to live. It's not a perfect choice, but at least it's our choice to make.

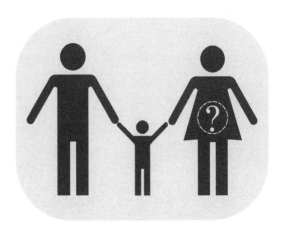

My Second Trimester

CHAPTER 12

faith and fiction

Amy: *Mattias, where does Santa Claus live?*

Mattias: *Oh, he lives in two stores.*

—Mattias, 3 years, 1 month

One of the worst things a parent can do is lose their child's trust and nothing will ensure that quicker than getting caught in a lie. Though not lying seems like a pretty clear-cut rule of parenting, sometimes it's not that simple.

I was driving around with Mattias in the back seat the other day when he asked me one of those questions I wasn't really prepared to deal with.

"Dad," he said, staring intently out the window, "is Santa Claus make-believe?"

"Where did you hear that?" I asked, trying to stall for time.

"Nowhere. I just wondered." He looked at me as if I was holding out, which I was. "So is he real or not?" I decided to lean on my old training from my educational consultant days, which taught me to answer every question with another question as often as possible.

"What do you think, buddy?" I felt like a psychoanalyst.

"Dad, just tell me." For a four-year-old, he has one hell of a bullshit detector.

"I think it's a pretty cool story, no matter what," I said, still dancing, "don't you?"

"Yeah," he said, "I like getting presents."

"Me too. Mommy and Daddy help out Santa with that kind of stuff, but it's up to you to decide how real you think Santa is." He went silent, which only happens if his wheels are turning quickly in that brain of his, or if he's unconscious. His eyes were open, so I knew he was rolling it around.

"OK," he said.

Whew. Glad to avoid a fit with a series of vague not-exactly-answers, especially in the car.

"What about Jesus?" he said, after a few moments of blessed silence.

"What about him?" I played dumb, waiting again to see what exactly I had to answer and what I could avoid.

"What about the stories about Jesus? Is he real?"

"Yeah," I sighed, growing increasingly anxious about dealing with this without my wife, the seminary graduate in the car. "Yeah, buddy, Jesus was real."

"He *is* real," Mattias corrected me.

"Well, he was alive a long time ago," I said.

"But they said at school and at church that Jesus is alive."

"Err, yeah," I hedged. "Sort of alive, I guess. Not really alive like you and me, exactly."

"How do you know?"

"I don't," I confessed. "It's just something I believe and that your mom believes."

"Why?"

Son of a toad-licker, why can't this car go any faster?

"Because," I said, picking my words carefully, "the way Jesus lived, the things he taught, and even the way he died are all the best examples we've ever found of how to be." I picked up the phone and dialed Amy, eager to be out from under the theological spotlight. Funny, how comfortable I am writing books and columns to thousands of people, and speaking to groups of hundreds about this stuff, while a kid who still wears pull ups at night can break me down to a heap of ignorance on a trip to the grocery store.

"Here," I said, handing the phone back to him, "ask your mom questions for a while."

I remember the exact moment when I found out Santa was not real, in the sense that I had previously thought he was real, anyway. It was Christmas Eve, of all days, and I was sitting on my aunt's lap in our townhome in Garland, Texas. My friends in the neighborhood, all of whom were older than I was, had teased me relentlessly for defending the existence of the fat man in red. I guess my folks finally decided enough was enough and that sending me back out to fight a specious battle was cruel and unusual.

Naturally, there were plenty of tears: mine, over the loss of a mythical figure I greatly admired, and my aunt's in commiseration over the loss of innocence. It didn't take long, though, until I started putting two and two together, leading me to ask about much more than I really wanted to know. Yes, the Tooth Fairy and the Easter Bunny are shams too. Damn, what a day.

"Do I still get my toys on Christmas?" I asked.

"Sure, you do."

"And candy on Easter."

"Yes, candy on Easter."

"OK," I conceded, "that's good." But then I started thinking about all the stories I had heard in church, and suddenly the miraculous stories about Jesus from the New Testament didn't seem much different than the legends about a fat man riding reindeer around the earth, stuffing himself down chimneys and giving away enough crap to equal the GDP of most countries.

This was one of the concerns I had even before Mattias was old enough to talk. I asked Amy her thoughts about doing the whole Santa Claus thing with our kids, in part because I knew how hard it could be to reconcile the dissolution of that concept some day with a faith you're supposed to hang on to throughout your whole life, yet with little more supporting evidence to go on. The other concern I had was more selfish, worried that once our kids figured out there was no actual Santa Claus, they would begin to doubt everything we had told—and would tell—them.

I don't want to raise cynical pragmatists any more than I want to set up my kids to be disillusioned by life at every turn. I do feel some responsibility to help him grow into some relationship with his faith as he ultimately defines it, but I also am less and less sure about what my job is in that respect.

For certain strains of Christianity, the rules are pretty clear. If you're Catholic, get your kid christened. If you're Protestant, the ultimate goal may be to keep your kid in church long enough to choose to be baptized, ensuring their hastening into the "good guys" category when that fateful day comes.

My less dogmatic take on belief doesn't make my job as parent any easier. I believe it's my responsibility to teach my kids to think on their own, to question, and I should make available to them a wide enough array of stories, beliefs, and historical perspectives that they can eventually arrive at their own conclusions. My own faith experiences aren't necessarily more "right" than someone else's. For a kid who, more or less, wants to know the rules of every game more than anything, this is not the kind of faith experience he's looking for right now.

The funny thing about religion is that each group is convinced they are right. If they don't, after all, why do they believe what they believe? For some, the differences among faiths are simply matters of personal experience, preference, or expression, whereas for others, they are defining lines in the sand that can be the distinction between infinite blessing and eternal damnation.

It will come as no surprise by now that I lean toward the former perspective more than the latter. There's an old allegory about a group of blind men and an elephant that best describes for me the human attempt to understand God. The first blind man goes up and grabs the elephant by the trunk and promptly proclaims to everyone he meets from then on that elephants are like serpents. Another feels the elephant's leg, which prompts him to describe the animal like a great oak tree. A third blind man, grabbing the elephant's tail, believes the elephant is like a rope and the final man, grasping the elephant's tusk, imagined the elephant as a long spear.

Are any of the men wrong? Would any of them agree about the nature of an elephant?

So who the hell am I, this relatively ignorant human being, groping around in the dark for God, having bumped into contact with some facet of what I consider to be divine, to be so arrogant and presumptuous as to try to teach another person about God?

I think the hardest part about it all for me with respect to faith and children is the sense of absolute trust and vulnerability they bring to you. Mattias would believe almost anything I told him, as long as I said it frequently and convincingly enough. I could probably set his mind on a course where the Flying Spaghetti Monster was the ultimate expression of God if I wanted to. That's a whole lot of power, and such power should be handled with tremendous care. With adults, you can share your own views, while trusting they will have the wherewithal to think for themselves and develop their own opinions. With kids though, they are tabula rasa, blank slates upon which you begin to etch your own understandings of reality, God, love, responsibility, truth, and evil. Some of that may be erased, rewritten, or otherwise recreated in time, but those first brush strokes are, in some ways, the most indelible.

In some ways, it's unfair to our kids that they're sort of bound to our particular church, at least until they have cars of their own or friends who can take them elsewhere to explore their faith. I enjoy talking to Mattias about the many varied faith traditions in the world, but at this point, those discussions are only substantial enough to show that our way of doing things is not the only way out there. In the meantime, it's my hope that we offer him the most positive, enriching, and loving image of God that we can, feeble old blind folks that we are.

This is not to say I don't have strong opinions though. He is currently going to a local Lutheran school because he missed the age cutoff for Kindergarten this year. It's connected to the Missouri Synod Lutherans, who are pretty conservative by Lutheran standards, and way far right of where I consider myself theologically. We chatted with the school leaders about their approaches, especially considering that the kids do daily Bible lessons and weekly chapel services. Assured that the focus is on Gospel messages of kindness, gentleness, and unconditional love, we decided to give it a try.

Things were pretty smooth for the first few days, at least until the first chapel service. During chapel, the pastor of the church led them in the Lord's Prayer, which we also say with Mattias at night before he goes to bed. Now there's a line that goes, "forgive us our sins, as we forgive those who sin against us." But there are lots of different versions of this part, replacing "sins" with "trespasses" or "debts." Well, Mattias is not exactly a lieutenant in the Dogma Police, but he does like things a certain way. We taught him the prayer using "sins," if for no other reason than it was the simplest word for him to say at the time. The pastor at his school, however, made the egregious error of using "trespasses."

"No!" hollered Mattias, right in the middle of the prayer, "It's sins, not trespasses!"

We heard about this one later.

I guess the pastor was fairly cool about it, and being a Missouri Synod Lutheran, he should be plenty comfortable arguing about dogmatic details like this. However, it may have been the first time he was ever corrected on his prayer language in the middle of a worship service, particularly by a four-year-old.

There were issues at his old school too, which was entirely nonreligious. One day, they apparently had crackers and grape juice as a snack, and he got into an argument with—of all kids—a Hindu classmate about whether or not their snack was actually the body of Jesus Christ.

We don't believe in the Catholic notion of transubstantiation, where the bread and wine actually become the body of Christ. For us, they are symbols only, but I guess symbolism is about as lost on a little guy as the idea of religious pluralism.

This sort of stuff cuts both ways though. Last week, he came home from school humming a song that sent shivers down my neck, though I wasn't sure why at first. Then he started signing the words, with great feeling:

I may never march in the infantry,
Ride in the cavalry, shoot the artillery,
I may never fly o'er the enemy,
But I'm in the Lord's Army!
YES SIR!

I know I said I'm all for him being exposed to a variety of religious ideas, but the notion of a paramilitary legion of preschool God Squadders makes me more than a little bit paranoid. Instead of freaking out, I just talked to him about what the song meant to him. I explained to him also that, although some people think of God that way, his mommy and I did not.

Two days later, he came home all excited about a story he had heard about this little kid named David killing a mean old giant bad guy with a slingshot. "He killed him dead, boy." He said confidently. "Goliath was bad, so David killed him with a rock, and God helped him do it."

"Now Mattias," Amy said, keeping the look of utter shock and disgust on her face concealed in the front seat of the car, "we don't kill people."

"Right," he said, smiling.

"Good," sighed Amy.

"Just bad people," he added.

"Monkey balls," I groaned under my breath. It reminded me of the when he came out of Children's church and proclaimed that God had killed thousands of Egyptians because people from Egypt are bad.

Ahh, how can words describe the pride I had at that moment for my blossoming little genocide-loving son?

"Yes, that story is in the Bible, isn't it?" I said after I gathered my thoughts.

"Yep," he grinned, "David killed lots of bad guys. Lots and lots of them."

"Yeah," I said, "right, wonderful. But just because something is in the Bible doesn't mean we do it, right?"

Silence.

"I mean," I continued, "you don't see me dragging you up a mountain, tying you to a rock, and trying to sacrifice you, do you?" I think the allusion to Abraham and Isaac was lost on him, but I was determined to make a point.

"No," he said sheepishly.

"And do we ever kill people? Good ones or bad ones?"

"No, we don't."

"That's right," I nodded, "and if we're not sure how to act sometimes, who is the best person to show us what the right choice is?"

"Jesus?" he raised his little eyebrows while staring at the passing scenery.

"I agree."

I was pretty proud of myself for redirecting the conversation without calling any of his teachers names I'd later regret. They have the best of intentions, I'm sure, but damn, sometimes people don't think about the way they teach these stories to kids.

Think about Noah and the ark. Sure, it's a cute story about rainbows, animals marching two-by-two, and God's mercy, right? But the subtext also is about the mass killing of most everything on the face of the earth.

Nighty, night, junior. Sleep tight and we'll see you in the morning, provided the waters don't rise in your sleep and engulf you in a watery grave. Don't let those bedbugs bite.

It seems kind of like we're using cutesy felt-board stories to water down the glorification of—or at least the justification for—violence. I'm not suggesting we avoid anything other than warm, fuzzy stories, but there's a level of discretion that should be used with certain ages. But sometimes we get so used to these old stories that we don't think anymore about how atrociously nasty parts of them really are, especially for literal-minded little children.

I have come to the conclusion that the best expressions of faith are not taught rhetorically anyway. Our kids learn more about loving our neighbors by watching us being loving toward them than by what we tell them. They learn about what's worth their time and energy by what we put our own time and energy into. It's disconcerting at best to think of this little person silently auditing my behavior, but that's part of what being a parent is about—making sure your walk matches your talk. It's great to talk about Jesus to your kids, but it's more important to *be Jesus* for them. Big shoes to fill, I know, but lots of people call God "Father" for a reason. Until they can understand the real one better, we're playing God in our kids' lives.

So do we keep putting the milk and cookies by the fireplace every year? Maybe I'll keep doing it, even if the kids couldn't care less.

CHAPTER 13

vagina nazis

My testicles are poofy.

—Mattias, 3 years, 1 month

We've officially moved from the "Whoopee, we're pregnant!" stage to the "you did this to me!" stage. For the most part, Amy has had a much easier pregnancy so far than she did the first time around, but there are these moments—these moments of gestational insanity, as I like to call them—when she temporarily loses her mind.

Leave it to me, of course, to jump in with my trademark pastoral point of view.

"Just remember," I said over coffee the other day, "when you want to pull a John Bobbitt on me in the middle of the night, that you're the one who wanted to do this."

"You guys get off so freaking easy," she snarled.

"Hey, I have to live with you," I said, sheepishly smiling after the words were already out there, hoping that she took it as a joke rather than a passive-aggressive swipe.

"I have to live with me too," she said, rifling through a bag of new stretchy pants and muumuu-style tops. "I hate being in the muffin top stage." This stage, in case you're not familiar, is when you're pregnant enough not to be able to fit into any of your old clothes, but not pregnant enough to actually look officially pregnant to the rest of the world. What you have instead is a belly that looks kind of like the top of a muffin that's baked over the edges of the pan.

Lucky for me she was too mired in self-loathing about her mutating body to be pissed off about my insensitive comments.

"Well, enjoy it," I said, stirring my coffee, "because this is the last round. Someone in this relationship will be sterile after this."

"It's gonna be you, pal," she said, which is only fair. But once again, I couldn't leave well enough alone.

"Hey," I said, "if they're already in there, they might as well tie off your plumbing. No reason to cut on my nuts unless absolutely necessary."

"How about we stop by the house and I go ahead and take care of it for you right now?" She was not amused. Fortunately, the old practice of always performing a cesarian section for every baby after you've had one C-section has gone by the wayside. Now you can delivery naturally, even if the first kid came out the emergency exit.

"I think I'll leave that one to the pros, thanks."

This week we have our first meeting with our midwife, or as I like to call her, the Vagina Nazi. I don't have much of a basis for my paranoia about meeting this woman, but I do recognize some wariness about going to meet with her.

It turns out that either some of the weird voodoo kind of stuff about midwives is either greatly exaggerated mythology or they've come a long way. Instead of having chicken bones and magic dust everywhere, this lady came in with a stethoscope and did her thing much like a regular physician. She even looked at me and shook my hand once Amy introduced me, which was nice. At first, I wasn't sure if I had put on my invisibility cloak or something, but contrary to popular belief, midwives do not have an insurmountable blind spot for all things testicular.

She got out this thing called a Doppler, which is a high-powered microphone to help you hear through uteruses. Even though we had seen the heart beat on the ultrasound before, it's altogether something else to hear it pumping away at about 160 beats a minute. I smiled like a proud daddy, while Amy cried—one of many such incidences for her throughout the day, by the way.

Have I mentioned how glad I am that guys can't get pregnant?

The midwife actually had some disappointing news for us. Obviously, in going with a midwife this time around, the goal was to deliver as naturally as possible. We based this hope mainly on the statistics we've seen in recent years about how many women have successfully delivered VBAC, or vaginal birth after C-section. It used to be that once a woman delivered by C-section, all subsequent births had to be done the same way. This had mainly to do with the fact that some women had problems with uterine ruptures while in labor, causing internal bleeding and other unpleasant stuff. But in the last couple of decades, C-sections have gotten to the point that they leave a lot less scarring, and thus reduce the risk of complications when doing a VBAC.

I guess we are just a couple of years too late to take advantage of this trend though. Given that we've become an obsessively litigious society, insurance companies, and subsequently, many hospitals, have told doctors that they will not cover doctors under their liability policies if they perform VBACs. This, unfortunately, was the case even for our midwife, whose insurance group has exerted the same pressure on her and her peers.

So basically, unless we go with a home birth, switch midwives, and pay for it all ourselves, we're most likely stuck with a C-section again. Though it's not a life-or-death issue, Amy took it pretty hard.

"It's terrible," said the midwife. "I've participated in more than a hundred VBAC births, all with no real complications, but now the business people have gotten involved, and what they say goes."

Putting myself in Amy's shoes for a minute, I was impressed she was only a little tearful. If someone I'd never met tried to tell me how I had to deliver my own child, I'd be wicked pissed. How messed up is it that our fear of risk has become such a fetish that we won't even let women choose how to deliver their babies? And how pathetic is it that hospitals bow to the pressure of the bottom line and let it happen? And although I can't absolutely say that Amy would not have had to have a C-section with Mattias if she had been allowed to go full term—keeping in mind that, although she wasn't due until the twenty-fourth, her doctor induced her on the nineteenth so he could go on vacation—I hold him partly to blame for the FUBAR situation we're in now.

What the hell—I've turned into a feminist . . .

There's the remote chance that one female doctor in the practice will still agree to do a VBAC, though it's not likely. After we got home last night, Amy mourned the loss of expectations of how this delivery might be different, and I basically sat there like a dip, not quite sure what to say. As she headed upstairs toward bed, I could hear her crying, partly because of pregnancy-related hormones, but also out of anger, disappointment, and even a little bit of grief, and I sat on the couch semiparalyzed by my inability to do much about it. In retrospect, I should have just gone upstairs, hugged her, and assured her that, no matter what happens, we'd be all right, and that the most important thing is her health and the baby's health, which no doctor or hospital would willfully compromise.

Instead I sat like a dork, reading my book about the Supreme Court until she quieted down and settled into sleep. The crying inflamed her sinuses so that she was snoring like a lumberjack by the time I got upstairs, which meant it was a night in the guest room for me.

Fair, enough, I thought to myself, my feet hanging off the end of the double bed, *this is what you get for doing nothing.*

I have never dealt well with strong emotions, whether they're coming from inside me or from someone else. Guys usually just want to "fix it," though one thing I've learned from having both a wife and a son is that tears don't necessarily mean something's broken. And sometimes the lack of emotions points to a bigger problem. Somewhere along the way, I learned—incorrectly—that feelings get in the way of life. Now that I'm surrounded by two of the more dramatic people I've ever known, I'm gradually coming to see it not only as acceptable, but even as strangely beautiful in how incredibly human it is.

That doesn't mean I don't keep trying to grab the emotional reins, mind you. It may be akin to trying to turn left while jumping off a cliff, but at least I find some consolation in the illusion that I'm in control.

CHAPTER 14

spawn of crazy

Amy: *Stay in your seat.*

Mattias: *Chicken feet.*

Me: *Mattias, sit down or you'll have to sit between us.*

Mattias: *Chicken penis.*

—Mattias, 2 years, 9 months

No one wants to have a crazy kid, but some of us are playing with a stacked deck. I'm one of those people.

So how stupid is it for someone who knows they have at least four consecutive generations of nuts on one side of his family alone to have kids? What sort of chance do they have? Though it might sound funny, this honestly was one of the biggest prohibitive factors for me about having kids at all, let alone two. I joke that the college fund we've set up for our kids can double as a therapy account, but I'd no sooner wish my experiences on them than I'd wish any other hell on earth. In some ways I'm lucky I even lived through it, so to put other people I love at risk by passing on my potential for craziness seems an unnecessary, if not foolish, risk sometimes.

Anyone who has made it this far realizes by now that my family has its share of eccentrics. Actually, we're probably not rich enough to be considered eccentric, but it sounds better than loony. I mentioned earlier that my great-grandmother shot herself in her garage and that my grandfather was the one who found her. Finding her is enough to mess up a kid for life, not to mention the fact that he inherited the same psychological issues that led my great-grandma to do that in the first place.

I didn't know my grandfather very well, and unfortunately, I learned more about him in the few months before he died than any other time in his life. In fact, the only time he ever told me he loved me was when he was lying on the couch in his living room, consumed by cancer and down to about eighty pounds. He held my little hand with the skeletal remains of his own and told me he loved me with the freedom of someone who finally had nothing left to lose.

It's strange to think about death as a liberating experience, but I think for my grandfather, whom we called Pop Pi, it was. My grandmother, Betty Piatt, had become known as "Pi" by her friends, and after a while it just stuck. Being the male counterpart, my grandfather naturally became Pop Pi. A World War II veteran, he had plenty of stories, most of which he rarely, if ever, cared to share. Most of the things I heard about him growing up were generally negative.

I know that, at one point, he moved from the family home in Kirkwood, Missouri, to Evansville, Indiana, to open a fried chicken restaurant. He had no previous experience in business ownership that I know of, and my dad often suspected he did it more out of an excuse to escape than to truly succeed as an entrepreneur, but the failure of the restaurant added to his bitterness nonetheless. I've also heard stories about how his nerves resulted in him being laid up in bed with stomach and back pains for weeks at a time, and there was apparently a year or more when he effectively relocated to the basement of the family house and rarely came out. To occupy himself, he read the entire encyclopedia from beginning to end, which points both to his intelligence and his lack of tolerance for normalcy.

I also learned, more than fifteen years after his death, that he was a fairly enthusiastic alcoholic. I never really noticed it myself, and we certainly never talked about it, but my mom brought up in conversation a couple of years ago that Pop Pi started each day with a screwdriver. Breakfast of champions, but only if you're trying to be Hunter S. Thompson. I'm not sure which is stranger: that he drank vodka for breakfast or that we never talked about it. Propriety was certainly a premium held in higher regard than open communication in the Piatt clan, which gives me more than a moment of pause in writing this book.

If there are two words my dad used more often than any others to describe Pop Pi, they were "bitter" and "angry." He used his thundering voice as a weapon, and used fear and intimidation to command order. Meanwhile, his internal chaos was an exact contradiction of the calm he tried to enforce around him.

My dad did much the same thing. He could make me cower with his baritone rants, and I learned all of my R-rated vocabulary well before making my way to kindergarten. If nothing else, I suppose I can thank him for that contribution to this project. He was an obsessive worker, staying at the office six or seven days most weeks, often ten to twelve hours a day or more. When he was home, he usually had ambitious remodeling projects to take on or a laundry list of errands to knock out. If he was home and sitting still, however, it was hardly an invitation to intimacy.

Off and on, my dad has been a smoker my whole life. He quit several times, but he's always gone back to it for one reason or another. I remember walking into the living room on weekends only to be slapped in the face by a dense cloud of cigarette smoke. It was really too much to handle, which was sort of the point, I think. My mom pointed out the construction of a fort-like barrier around himself that he'd generally create too with his stack of papers and magazines on one side and a row of potato chip bags and candy jars on the other.

Though my dad rarely, if ever, kicked off the day with a cocktail, I can't say that his morning diet of chips, candy, and soda were a particularly healthier alternative. His eating habits were another barrier that was hard for folks to overcome, serving as an excuse many times not to attend certain social events and also to command control over our household.

These barriers were everywhere. When not literal, like the candy and paper fortress, the walls were composed of obsessive busyness and a tireless work ethic. The result of his obsession was, in some ways at least, fruitful. He made a buttload of money in the eighties as an insurance salesman, rising to the top of his large international company. He won trips all over the world and garnered praise and admiration from his peers. The problem was, when he came home, he was "just" a dad and a husband, which seemed to suffocate him.

For a while, my mom worked at my dad's agency, possibly with the hope of giving them some common thread to hold them together. I would call most days after school and ask her if he was in a good enough mood to say "hi," which I only learned later was a strange dynamic for a father and son. If he did happen to answer the phone himself, I could tell within a handful of words how the conversation was going to go.

On the upside, living with such a volatile and unpredictably angry person makes for wonderfully codependent kids. I was a pro at molding myself around his moods and only later did I decide that having to tiptoe through my whole life was bullshit, though that brought a host of other problems along with it.

For years, I had dreamed of my parents getting a divorce. A lot of my friends' folks had split, so I figured it was just some whim of mine to fit in with them, kind of like wishing for braces or glasses just to be a little bit different. But in time, I realized this longing for them to go their separate ways actually was a pretty accurate barometer for the health of their relationship, independent of me. They told me, some years after they actually divorced midway through my senior year in high school, that they stayed together longer than they might have "for me." Well, thanks, but no thanks. It wasn't that great staying together just for the sake of sticking it out.

I give my parents points for trying, though. Our family didn't disintegrate until after a healthy dose of therapy. We tried pretty much every combination, including individual, marriage, and family shrinks. My adventure into the Freudian Froot Loop world began with my school counselor, who my folks asked to visit with me after my grades started to slip. Admittedly, I was pissed, but this had more to do with frustration about my family life, a private all-boys school I was rebelling against, and general teenage hormonal insanity than anything else.

Still, when she'd ask me questions, I'd answer honestly. After all, I had no reason not to trust her. After a few weeks, she did a few tests with me, including the interminable MMPI (Minnesota Multiphasic Personality Inventory), which has more questions than my four-year-old son, and the Rorschach inkblot test. I gave them all my best shot, though now I wish I had taken what I like to call the "Keith Olberman" approach. Precocious and pretty tough to handle during his school age years, his parents had him tested too, with the same tests, in fact. But instead of cooperating, every time they'd show him another inkblot, he'd say, "It looks like an inkblot," and nothing else.

Man, to have that opportunity back and drop a gem like that . . .

I guess I didn't give the right answers, because the next thing I knew, I was shipped off to meet a couple of times a week with this arrogant shrink who I'll call Dr. Outlaw. That's not his real name, but several civil cases later his actual moniker is just as darkly ironic. Anyway, I didn't know much about this new shrink, except that he came across as a real schmuck sandwich, and for some reason, I was just supposed to start spilling my guts to him as soon as I met him. Truth is, I liked my school counselor as much as I hated Dr. Outlaw, and I resented having no say in whom I talked to, so more often than not I just didn't talk much.

That turned out to be a bad idea.

It turns out that, if your dad is an insurance agent and your shrink is one of the admitting doctors for one of the biggest local adolescent psychology wards, you should answer any questions they throw at you. One Saturday afternoon my folks told me that we were going on a day trip, which sounded good enough to me. But instead of heading out of town, we went straight to Outlaw's office. In the parking lot, my dad popped the trunk and pulled out a suitcase, this made me sweat a little but there wasn't much I could do at the moment except go along. Once in the doctor's office, they told me they were bringing a "nurse" from the unit across the street to take me over and admit me to the loony bin.

Now when you picture a nurse, you probably have the same image that I do, but this dude was anything but that. He was more like a bouncer than a nurse, which was when I realized they had been lying to me about this whole process because they considered me a "flight risk," meaning they figured I would have run away if I'd known about their plans ahead of time. They may have been right, but no matter how you cut it, it completely sucks to be tricked into getting locked up.

I was told I'd go over to this unit for a two-week assessment, which I assumed meant I'd only be there for two weeks. But when I told the kids in my first group session that, they all howled with contempt. They started rattling off their sentences for me: six months, eighteen months, three years.

I felt like I was going to puke.

For the first few days I had to live in what was called the Day Room, which was the big meeting area in front of the main desk. The unit was locked off with electromagnetically sealed doors and the windows were tinted dark and covered with thick security wire. After taking all of my jewelry and shoelaces away, they explained to me that my unit was on "lockdown," which basically meant they weren't getting along the way the docs in charge felt like they should. As a consequence, there were a few restrictions on everyone for the whole time I was there, including no television, no radio or any other music, no magazines or newspapers, and no going outside. Twenty-four hours of every day were spent behind the locked doors of the unit, which actually was better than some kids had it.

They did pair us up once I got to stay in an actual room, so we had at least a little bit of company. My first roommate was Dave, and he was a crazy bastard. He had fried his nut one time too many doing acid, and most of the time he just talked about the band Motorhead. We each had days assigned when we could do laundry and everyone on that day had to negotiate taking turns with the two machines we had. Todd, not exactly the brightest light on the porch, would wander down the hall and when he inevitably found the machine was being used, he'd bring all of his stuff back to the room instead of queuing up to wait his turn.

He didn't finally get his chance that day until after dinner, but when he went down to start his load, the staff told him it was too late and that he'd have to wait another week. He was understandably pissed and came back into the room grumbling obscenities under his breath. He slammed his bag of laundry down on his bed, which made enough of a racket to bring the nurse who had followed him down the hall into our room. Without another word, he grabbed his walkie-talkie and radioed for backup.

A minute later, we heard the worst two words to hear on our unit come over the loudspeaker: Doctor Rush.

This was code for an out-of-control kid who needed to either be sedated, restrained, or both. Within a few minutes, six men came in with straps and cuffs and secured him to the bed. This, Dave noted, was hardly the first time it had happened to him, but it may have ended up being his longest stint. They didn't let him loose from that godforsaken bed for nearly four weeks. He had to piss in a bedpan, eat in bed, and even get spongebaths, which wouldn't have been so bad if the one administering them hadn't been the same bouncer-nurse that helped admit me.

More than two months into my stint, I was crawling the walls. I hadn't seen the light of day all summer, and with a robust insurance policy backing my stay, there was no end in sight. It was only after my parents finally threatened Dr. Outlaw that he conceded to let me continue my "treatment" in a day program, which was where I spent the next six or eight months.

I felt somewhat vindicated a few years later when the facility where I was held and several of the doctors involved with it were slapped with multiple accusations of fraud and other criminal nonsense. I found great pleasure in watching the hospital eventually turned into a pile of rubble, though Outlaw got to continue practicing.

I'm not going to suggest that I was the picture of mental health back in those days, but given the fact that my folks divorced less than a year after I underwent treatment would suggest that there was a whole lot more going on than just the problems I had as a rebellious teenager. In fact, I went on to finish high school at an arts school in downtown Dallas, and my college years at the University of North Texas were some of the best of my life. It wasn't until after college that I had my full-on breakdown, which might suggest my shrinks were about seven or eight years premature in their original work with me.

I won't go into the gory details, but for those of you who can relate to the so-called dark night of the soul, that time in my life certainly was mine. I heard voices, holed up in my room, and drank so much many nights that I don't remember where I was. I'd go to see Doc, my still-friend and mentor, especially since he'd see me for free when I had no money, which was often. However the psychotropic drugs back then were not nearly as good as they are now and they had pretty debilitating side effects. There are chunks of months that I honestly don't remember at all from my twenties, though some of the friends I had back then whom I still keep in touch with now will tell you I was a different person.

At the risk of product placement, I should mention that Prozac rocks my gonads off. It has been the answer for me, along with years of what I call "real" therapy, a hell of a lot of personal will, and both a faith and family that have shown me a different reality. My life is hardly perfect.

One of the reasons I love Amy so much is that she sees dimensions of me that I don't, or perhaps won't, see. Where I find weakness and instability, she sees the strength of someone who has overcome incredible challenges. When I wrestle with fits of inadequacy, she reminds me of the goodness she sees. And in those times when I get bogged down in obsessive fretting about our kids' fates, she urges me to watch my son, who is the embodiment of joyful living in the moment, spreading his lust for life like a virus to everyone he meets.

His life does help remind me that even the worst of conditions can produce incredible things like him. He's a walking, talking miracle if I've ever seen one, and although his life won't be perfect by any means, the world is a better place for having him in it. For all I know, the next kid could be a poop-slinging nutjob, but we don't have kids because we're guaranteed the results we want. We have them because the love contained within us longs to be expressed.

The risk of investing your heart in another person, whether you grew them or not, borders on insanity in itself, but if what I lived through growing up was the bad kind of crazy, I think it's safe to say that family life is, on most days at least, a pretty good kind of crazy.

CHAPTER 15

who's your daddy?

*Dad, I love you and you love me, and even when you're
mad, you love me too.*

—Mattias, 3 years, 0 months

There's a social phenomenon I like to call the Jerry Springer Effect. I've watched a few minutes here and there of shows like Springer and they all pretty much make me want to take a shower. They piss me off and generally feed my misanthropic inclinations, which don't need any help making me jaded about the future of the human race.

The only thing I can figure out about why people watch shows like Springer and reality court television shows is because the losers on those shows make people feel better about themselves. No matter how bad your life is, you can always plop down for some midafternoon entertainment and a bag of chips and stuff your face while shaking your head in contempt.

"At least I'm not that guy," you may say to yourself. Well, if you're sitting around watching Jerry Springer and eating Ho-Hos, you're not very far from it.

My point isn't to bitch about television though. It's that this so-called art actually reflects life in a perverse sort of way. Every once in a while, when I'm walking around Pueblo, I feel like Jim Carey in *The Truman Show*, except instead of being plopped down in the middle of my own reality show, I've taken a left turn into a *King of the Hill* episode with more brown people.

There are plenty of great people in Pueblo, even if the average fashion sense got a blowout some time around 1986 and hasn't progressed since. But mullets, lower back tattoos, sleeveless T-shirts, and giant bangs thankfully don't reflect on the person underneath it all.

Unfortunately though, we also have a disproportionate share of crappy parents. Given some arm's-length objectivity, it can make you feel pretty good about yourself, just feeding and bathing your kid every day. And if you are still married and both parents are living together under the same roof, you're way ahead of the curve. It's not like this trend is unique to Pueblo. Grandparents raising their grandchildren, single moms trying to piece together a life for their kids on minimum wage and public assistance, kids giving birth to kids, and so on. It's particularly obvious in our community, with our high dropout rates, high teen pregnancy, and robust gang involvement, but crappy parenting knows no social class or ethnicity.

While the two-job, gold-collar family may provide their kids with more stuff, they can suck at being parents far worse than a couple in the ghetto. To paraphrase an old cliché, any loser with a penis can be a father, but it takes a special man to be a dad.

I used to work in some of the poorest public schools in town, where I witnessed the kind of neglect and abuse these eight- and nine-year-old kids endured. We've had families in our own church damaged and even broken by addiction, and the kids look like they've been through combat. And guess who's most likely to follow in mommy's and daddy's footsteps? After all, where else do they learn more about what it means to be an adult?

There are a handful of men in the African-American community who have broken popular silence and spoken out against the inferior parenting job of their fellow black men. Public figures like Bill Cosby, Juan Williams, and Barack Obama have taken more than a small amount of heat for their directness too, but at least they're getting the dialogue started. Are we really as crappy at parenting as these guys are saying? Are we doing anything about it?

It would be easy enough to sit back and blame our parenting crisis on black men, or on poor people, or on anyone other than ourselves, but if there's a kid in our community who is suffering from an absence of a decent role model, what the hell are we waiting for?

Beyond that, what the hell makes any of us qualified to be parents? As for Amy and me, we joke sometimes that with seven marriages between our four parents, we know at least a little bit about what to try to avoid. But the reality is that, no matter how many books we read and no matter how hard we try, we're going to screw up our kids.

Happy parenting!

But let's at least get it out on the table. You, I, and everyone else who squeezes out a kid will, without question, do something to screw them up. Many somethings, most likely. Some of us will screw up our kids beyond repair, while others may have the awareness and resources to get our kids into counseling, even before they leave home, with the hope of maybe un-screwing them up. Whatever your upbringing though, and no matter how much money you make or how many Baby Einstein DVDs you buy, your kids have a 100 percent chance of getting screwed up and you'll be the one who did it.

How do we make up for it? I believe by resolving never to look at someone else's situation and say to ourselves, possibly with some relief, that it's not our problem.

Children never were meant to be raised alone, by two people sequestered away in a suburb somewhere. Tribal parenting is in our genetics, and our obsession with privacy and personal success—mine included, mind you—has cut us off from the sources of support that are supposed to naturally be there to help us raise kids.

Because guess what? Raising kids is hard work. And none of us knows how to do it entirely alone.

We were giving a couple of kids from our church a ride to a summer day camp with Mattias, because their folks aren't involved, and I don't mean just with church. These two boys are a couple of the cutest kids on the planet, which is a good thing for them because they can both be real Grade-A pains in the ass.

We were driving back from the camp when the two boys—we'll call them Spongebob and Patrick—start going at each other.

"Your dad's in jail," said Patrick, who is four years old.

"Shut up," scowled Spongebob, who is six.

"He don't love you," grinned Patrick, Spongebob's cousin. They live under the same roof though, for the life of me, I could not plot their family tree or who actually lives in the house, even with the help of NASA.

"You shut up, stupid," Spongebob was getting pissed.

"Hey," Mattias said, "that's not nice. Be kind and loving to each other." I felt proud that he had the confidence and an affirming enough childhood to date to speak up, but I also was a little bit sad about how incredibly naive he sounded. The world is going to kick my kid in the junk more than once.

"He's in jail," Patrick crooned, "your dad's in jail."

"Spongebob," Amy said in her best, most soothing Martha Stewart voice, "your daddy loves you no matter what. Even if he's not around, he still loves you."

"No, he don't!" The two boys started punching each other.

"Oh, yes he does," Mattias sat up. "He loves you even if you make bad choices. There's nothing you can do to make your dad stop loving you."

"We love you too, buddy," I said to Spongebob, trying to act like some sort of role model in the two or three minutes we had left before we dropped them off.

"No you don't," Spongebob shouted. Little tears were gathering in the corners of his eyes. "Y'all don't love me. I'll just die and be a ghost."

"Then I guess we'd love your ghost," I said, shrugging my shoulders, trying not to give him the reaction he was looking for.

"I'd scratch you all up and eat you."

"I guess we could love you as ghost food," I said, turning to Amy, "what do you think?"

"Sure, why not?"

"I hate this stupid car," he glared, "and I hate you and I hate that church and I'm never, ever going back. I'm just going to die and never come back."

The fact that any six-year-old kid can ever have the experiences to draw on for such anger, despair, and hopelessness should be criminal.

"You know what," I said, turning around in my seat and looking him in the eye, "it's fine if you're mad. It's fine if you cry or if you don't want to talk at all. But you don't use words like 'stupid' in our family. I don't want to hear it again. Understand?"

Well, that did it. The dam broke and just as we pulled up in the driveway of their house, of course.

"You're a big meanie," he wailed, pulling at the car door handle. "I don't want to see you ever again." He ran toward the porch, then threw himself down on the front step where I was sure to see him crying and he could watch my reaction while he put on his little show. I waved at him as we pulled out and turned away.

"See you Sunday," I said out the window and we were gone.

Sure enough, Sunday came around, and Spongebob and Patrick among the first ones to show up. They started playing right away with Mattias and came over a couple of times to show me some random pieces of crap they found in the carpet. Then their aunt came over to me and I was ready to get an earful. I could only imagine, with Spongebob's propensity for lying, what he had told her and his mom about me. I mean, it took us three days into the camp just to figure out how old he really was. So even though his aunt was a diehard friend, I cringed a little as she came my way.

"Did the boys give you an earful on the way over?" I asked.

"Yes, they did," she smiled, "but they always do."

"Did they mention our last day together this week?"

"No, but when they got in the car, they asked me where we were going and I told them we were going to learn about the best person in the whole world. And Spongebob perked up and said, 'Oh, we're going to see Mattias's dad?' Just thought you'd like to know I guess you're on up there in his book with the Big Guy."

Well, go figure.

Turns out that little seeds aren't so hard to plant in kids' lives. You may never personally know if they ever bear fruit or what kid of fruit they bear even if they do, but resolving to plant them anyway, no matter how rocky and unforgiving the soil, is in itself an act of love.

For the most part, Spongebob and Patrick's lives still suck, but at least if they live long enough to reflect on it they'll remember that at least some little parts of the world might not be quite as bad as they thought. Call me an idealist, but I have to believe that encounters like these can change a life. I'm not saying it's guaranteed, but with a little luck and maybe some divine providence, I hold on to the hope that these kids, and millions of others like them, will have the chance to learn that ultimately love wins.

CHAPTER 16

sleep drought

Grandma *Suzie: Mattias, did you have good dreams last night?*

Mattias: *I had a good dream and a bad dream, but the bad dream broke the good dream.*

—Mattias, 3 years, 4 months

Sleep is a funny thing; you feel like you can't function without it, but I've never known of anyone who has died from lack of it. Of course, it messes up your body, but somehow no matter how little you get your system finds a way to push through.

It's a good frigging thing or all toddlers would be orphans.

I'm not a big fan of all the scare tactics people throw at you when you decide to have kids. "Oh, you think they're tough as newborns? Wait 'till they're two." Then you finally learn first-hand why they call it the Terrible Twos and some sphincter pronounces that three is way worse than two ever was, just wait.

There's some weirdness to how the whole system works. When you meet someone, everybody immediately wants to know when you're going to get engaged. When you finally do, and if you ever talk to them about the challenges of adjusting to such a major commitment, all they want to do is tell you how much harder actually being married is. Once you're married, everybody's in your business about when you're going to have kids. Then as soon as you're finally pregnant, they give you one of the "Oh, just wait" lectures. You know what I'm talking about.

"You think morning sickness is tough now? Oh, just wait until you're the size of a special-ed school bus and you need a front-end loader to roll over in bed."

"You think the first year of marriage is challenging? Oh, just wait until this kid is born. You'll never wet your wiener again."

"You think you aren't getting much sleep with one kid? Just wait until you have another one. Speaking of, when are you kids going to start trying for the next one?"

Bite me.

This ceaseless back-and-forth between questions about what you're going to do next, followed by proclamations of how bad it's going to suck once you do, is enough to make a guy want to hole up in a cave with a Playboy and a bag of Cheetos.

Marriage is great but it's also hard. Most things that are worthwhile are. Same goes with kids. There are days when you can't imagine the world without them, and then there are others when you wonder how much they'd sell for by the pound on the black market.

This weekend, we had one of those days. Technically, it was just a night I guess, but it spilled over into the next day. The shockwave effect of sleep deprivation is awesome.

We had some friends come into town to spend the night after a concert they put on. They have two kids, one of whom is a nine-year-old girl named Brianna and the other is a five-year-old boy named Devin, who gives Mattias a run for his money. I'm not going to say the kid is loud, but he's certainly got the pipes for opera if he ever decides to lean that way.

Mattias pretty much lost his shit, as he is prone to doing when kids spend the night. Now that we've demolished one of our guest bedrooms by making it into a bathroom, we only have one bedroom left for guests. So to let the kids have some time to goof around while their folks had some privacy, we put all three of them in the same room together. Devin slept in the bed with Mattias while Brianna slept on an air mattress on the floor.

How she slept through all the ridiculous events that night, I'll never know. I envy her sleeping prowess.

One thing to keep in mind is that we live in a house built in 1901. We had something called a swamp cooler, which circulates water through these filters then sucks air through them and blows it through the house. Basically, it's a half window unit that's supposed to cool down the whole house, and it only does this very well in the summer if you leave it on all the time.

The problem is that it's located in the guest room, so they either leave the swamp cooler on and freeze to death or we all drown in pools of sweat as the radiant heat from the day seeps in from the outside bricks. It's basically like sleeping in an oven turned on low heat for about eight hours.

Our houseguests, not aware that this was the only source of air for everyone, shut the thing off before they went to sleep. It started heating up within half an hour or so, but there was nothing to do without waking them up and freezing them out so we just dealt with it. The problem was that Mattias is a hot sleeper as it is, but with another little heat generator sleeping next to him, those two put out enough BTUs to power the whole house.

So Mattias woke up about three in the morning, first to pee, but also to try to cool down. Amy got up first with him, which he saw as the perfect opportunity to work an angle.

"I want to sleep with you," he said. "It's hot in there." The problem was, it was hot everywhere and by now we're all up—all except for the guests that is, who seem to be sleeping through everything blissfully. Mattias loves to try to work it so he can end up in our room but I can't handle more bodies in my bed. First of all, I don't like anything touching me when I'm sleeping, including Amy. We have a king-size bed for a reason. Even though he's a little guy, Mattias is kind of like helium; he'll take up as much room as you give him. If you can get some shut-eye while someone is simultaneously kneeing you in the balls and drooling on your pillow, it's a great system, but otherwise you need to keep your kids in their own room.

Some parents seem not to mind having their kids in their bed with them. I think they're masochists. Aside from the violence a thrashing kid exacts on you, on top of the incredible heat they put off, you'll never cha-cha again with kids in and out of your room all night. That's enough right there to put the kibosh on kids in bed for me.

So back to the hallway debate about where he'd sleep. I've figured out that if I ever want to get something from Amy really badly, I should wake her up after about three hours of sleep, drag her out in the hallway, and ask her. She's a total pushover. Instead of sending him back to his room and risking a conflict that might wake everyone up, she conceded and let him into our room. Problem was, I was not about to give up on the rest of my own sleep. Just because she can conk out while being judo kicked in the skull doesn't mean I want to put up with it.

"Come here, boy," I said, squinting into the hallway light. He started to try to edge around me to make it over to his mom's side of the bed where he knew he'd be in safe territory.

"No," he scowled. "Mommy said I can sleep with her."

"I said come here," I grabbed for him and pulled him to the edge of the bed, which promptly sent him into a tailspin.

"Daddy pulled me!" he wailed at the top of his lungs. "He's mean. He grabbed me! Oweeee!" Lights started turning on in the guest room, but once they poked their head out and saw it wasn't their kids, they rolled back over and went back to sleep. Had I been more clear-headed, I would have asked them to turn the swamp cooler back on, but I was too busy wrangling a freaking-out kid while half asleep.

"God, honey," Amy sighed, "you're just making it worse."

"He is not sleeping in here," I said.

"Mommy, daddy's grabbing me!" Mattias howled.

"You're going to wake up everyone in the house."

"Really?" I snapped. "Do you hear me crying at the top of my lungs?"

"Let me go!!!" He hollered. By now I was wide awake and seething.

"You have five seconds to get your butt back in that bed of yours," I sat up, "or I'll haul you in there myself."

"Really nice," Amy grumbled.

"I didn't ask for parenting advice." Did I mention our worst arguments happen in the middle of the night when we get woken up unexpectedly?

"I didn't see you get up with him," she said. "I'm the one who got up, not you."

"Well I'm up now and I'm dealing with it, so back off."

"You're being mean to mommy."

"Everybody shut up," I snarled. "You have three seconds."

Mattias squealed in anger as he sprinted to his room, tripped over Brianna sleeping at the foot of his bed, crawled over Devin, and buried his head in his pillow, crying. His two guests didn't so much as roll over through the whole thing.

By the time I took a leak, grabbed some water, and got back in bed, I was so pissed off I couldn't think straight let alone try to sleep. Mattias fell back asleep, amazingly within ninety seconds or so, which made me even more envious that he could stir up so much drama and then pass out while I'm still swimming in the aftermath. I knew I'd been an ass to Amy, but the last thing I feel like doing when I'm angry is apologize, so I laid there for a good hour or so, thinking of all the wry comebacks I could shoot her way if she dared to try to talk to me.

As he tends to do, Mattias woke up the next morning all smiles and I dragged myself toward the coffee pot. I mustered enough energy to see our guests off while Mattias played on his keyboard, apparently oblivious to the previous evening's conflict. Had he already forgotten? Was he sleepwalking through the whole thing?

It's funny, because as short as the emotional fuses are of little kids, their emotional memory banks are equally short-lived. I've seen Mattias throw such a raging fit that he's almost made himself vomit, and within twenty minutes he's laughing and playing like it never happened. The parents are the ones who seem to have a harder time letting go. I play the whole thing over and over again in my head, thinking about how I might have handled things differently without the handicap of sleep to contend with. Amy and I both talked through it easily enough that morning, but I was left not only with a sleep deprivation hangover, but also an emotional rawness that put me on edge for most of the day.

Thankfully Mattias still takes naps on the weekends, and I didn't have any commitments later that day, so we all crashed hard after lunch. By the time we finally roused ourselves, all was right with the world and we went and had some fun at the park.

Parenting, if done well, is one of the most selfless acts in humankind. The problem is that, no matter how hard we try to put our spouse, our children, or even our principles as parents before ourselves, we all have at least one Achilles's heel. For me it's sleep, as if that wasn't already abundantly obvious. For others it may be something else, but anyone, no matter how much I love them, who gets between me and a good night's rest is setting themselves up for problems.

It's in moments like those when I realize how basically animalistic I still am. It's not so much that we ever get over our animal nature, but rather we learn how to attenuate it and set aside our more self-centered impulses for the betterment of the group. But there are moments for each of us when the social conscience takes a backseat to the "me first" beast. I'm not crazy about it, and most people never even see it, but unfortunately the ones who suffer the ill effects of this side of me are the ones I love the most. It's hardly fair, but it's definitely the "worse" part of the whole "for better or worse" vow you make when you take the plunge of marriage.

Kids, on the other hand, don't have a choice. We didn't call a little family meeting with the sperm and egg in question before making a kid; we just did it and here he is. I still resent the negative impact his behavior has on me sometimes, or on our marriage, but hell it could be argued I had a pretty big impact on his state of affairs. He didn't get to choose his parents or where he lives. We try to give him some agency over daily choices like the clothes he wears and what snack he wants, but for the most part everything in his world is decided for him.

It's a delicate balance, giving him enough latitude to make his own choices while also looking out for both his best interest and preserving the needs I have as an individual and as a husband. I get why he wants to sleep with us, but he simply has to get that need for being close to us met in another way. It means I have to make more time in our waking hours to meet that need. But that doesn't make it any easier to deal with him at the moment he's trying to crawl into bed when I'm bleary-eyed from lack of sleep.

It's an imperfect system, and I'll never claim to be the perfect parent, but at the very least I try to learn enough from the traumatic events to avoid—or at least mitigate—them the next time around.

Chalk up at least one lesson learned from the whole night; we've since decommissioned the swamp cooler and placed an air conditioner in the hallway. This in itself doesn't make me a better parent, but I'm hoping it at least gives me fewer opportunities to be a crappy one.

CHAPTER 17

lightning strikes

(After the lights went out during a storm)

Amy: *No! Come on!*

Mattias: *Mommy's mad at the electricity.*

—Mattias, 2 years, 9 months

The same afternoon we had our latest ultrasound, lightning struck the steeple at the Catholic church down the street. I'm not saying the two are connected, but if you're one for omens something like that will get your attention.

After months of little or no rain, we made up for most of the drought in one afternoon yesterday. The storm first rolled in from Beulah, up in the mountains where I've been doing some work, and it followed me all the way back to Pueblo. I could tell from the dark, angry swell of the clouds that we were going to get hammered.

The coffee shop downtown where Amy and I were hanging out lost their power, so we sat in the dark and enjoyed the sound of the rain. Located in a retrofitted garage, the coffee shop is not exactly waterproof and the staff would come out from behind the counter every few minutes to mop up the water oozing in from under the rolling doors and floor-level portal windows.

While we were sitting in the dark, a series of lightning bolts hit close enough to rattle the window panes. We were about two miles from home, and it had clearly made contact somewhere between the coffee shop and our place. We learned later, and saw for ourselves as we drove by, that it had hit the steeple of one of the local Catholic churches, called the Cathedral of the Sacred Heart. And even though a basic lesson in physics can explain the strike—the steeple, at 130 feet, is one of the highest points in town, topped off with a big metal cross at the point—the superstition of the locals was rampant within hours of the event.

The steeple caught fire and although I'm only sure of one lightning strike, we heard that while the firefighters were putting out the first blaze, a second bolt hit at the very same spot. Of course, people were quick to say that this was God's way of getting the church's attention for recent indiscretions, both nationally and locally too. Onlookers wondered aloud if Bishop Tafoya was taking notes or if he was hiding under a table somewhere, hoping not to be the next on God's hit list.

Personally, I don't believe in a God that doles out punishment in such a manner. I mean, lightning bolts? There are those who suggest that disasters such as the AIDS pandemic, the floods in New Orleans, and earthquakes in China are divine payback for the wrongs of humanity, but honestly I think we humans do a pretty good job of screwing ourselves up without God's help.

There have been times when I watch Mattias about to do something really stupid and instead of stopping him, I'll let him go ahead and do it just to let him learn firsthand what the consequences of his behavior can be like. I don't really consider God to be this human-like parent so much as a cosmic creative force or impetus, but if God has such things as will and force, I also believe that God exercises restraint at least in equal measure.

I should also mention that the same church burned down some 125 years ago, which adds to the bad mojo around it. Whether God did it or not, I suppose that any act of nature that leads people to reflect on their lives, both individually and collectively, is a good thing.

In reality, the bad press the Catholic Church has received on a local level happened a long time ago, although it lingers like a sort of bad hangover; the kind you get once you reach thirty-five and you only have three beers, but forget your aspirin and extra glass of water before bed. Despite public apologies from the diocese, the stories of a local priest who worked in an area high school and systematically drugged and molested one boy after another in the supply closet hang around like a dark cloud.

There are a couple of reasons why this kind of thing is hard to let go. As a person of faith, I can understand how betrayed someone feels, not only by the priest himself who carried out this horrific behavior for years on end, but also the greater church who transferred him once the story broke but did not keep him from being a priest. It's a sign of a broken system and one that sometimes puts people and agendas before principles. It's discouraging, but in the end the church is a human-made and human-run system. No matter how much we pray, how hard we work, or how much we hope, it will fail us sometimes.

As a parent, my paranoia rises when I think of the implicit trust between a minister and a child. Who the hell can you trust if your pastor may be diddling your son in the rectory? It's one way in which Amy's gender can actually be an asset in her profession, whereas often it's a liability in some peoples' eyes. At least, people figure, my kids are safe with a woman. Though this isn't a guarantee either, the perception of the sexual predator rightfully falls more often on men's shoulders.

It's all enough to make me want to lock my kids in their room until I arrange a marriage and send them off to live happily ever after.

All of this is swirling around in my head as we go in for the ultrasound. Here's this persistent little heartbeat, plugging away at 140 beats a minute in my wife's abdomen. Aside from it being really freaky to hear a heartbeat coming from a person's stomach, it's yet another reminder of the incredible vulnerability of life. After checking the heartbeat they send us upstairs for blood work, which will indicate whether or not there are any number of birth defects likely.

I call this the Baby Dud test.

I let Mark, Amy's dad, know that if this baby's a dud, we'll just send it to live with him. That's his payback for pushing us to procreate and then putting his pastoral powers of prayer to work for triplets.

Anyway, it's been my position that for a baby to qualify as a dud, it would just have to be obnoxious, eat too much, not let me sleep when I want, or something like that. But going through the litany of possible maladies they were testing for gives a worry-prone parent all kinds of new things to obsess about for the next week until the results come back. To relieve some of my own anxiety, I called Mark and let him know he'd find out in a week or so if he was going to be a new daddy.

Some people argue that such tests are pointless, especially if you're not planning to terminate the pregnancy if the tests come back with bad news. We're resolved to keep the baby no matter what, but there's an argument to be made for knowing ahead of time if complications may arise. First off, there are actually some surgeries that can be performed now in utero to correct problems of an unborn fetus. If I can do something even before the kid is born to ensure the most normal possible life, I'm all for it. Also given the fact that we only have two modest hospitals in town here, it would be good to know if we should plan to deliver somewhere that might be better prepared for things like a heart condition or the like.

As I've mentioned before though, there are no guarantees, even if the baby has all ten fingers and toes and everything seems normal. Life is a gamble. It's risky business, made even more treacherous with every person you depend on. Granted, it's also made more full in the same way, but loving other people, I've found, is a little bit like a running around in a storm with a lightning rod.

Ministry is one of those vocations where you can't help but see on a daily basis how often, and how hard, lightning can strike the human condition. I drove Amy to a local shelter where folks from our congregation serve dinner once a month. It's a relatively small gesture to someone whose life has effectively been destroyed, but it's at least an acknowledgement of their existence. It also keeps us from letting ourselves off the hook, pleading ignorance about how things really aren't so bad, and therefore we don't really have too much work to do.

It doesn't, however, keep me from being a selfish, greedy, self-centered bastard. We were sitting outside the shelter, waiting for her fellow servers to show up, when we started talking about a recent book manuscript of mine. I got word that a publisher who has been sitting on my novel for six months showed a promising step in their review process. Nothing's a guarantee in the book world, but when you're waiting months on end for any interest, the smallest gesture will start your imagination spinning.

"If I sell this book," I said, "I want to get something cool."

"Like what?" Amy asked. I said nothing. "You're not getting a scooter," she said.

"Dammit." She's psychic or something.

"Maybe you could get a new TV."

"Nah," I shook my head, "you'd like that too much. I want to get something cool that you don't want."

"Really nice."

"Well, I wrote the book," I protested. "I should get something cool."

"You deserve something cool?"

"I don't know, but I want it."

"Want what?" she turned toward me.

"I dunno," I shrugged. "Something cool. And something that you don't want."

"You're a goof." We sat silently as the rain trickled down the windshield. I could tell that she was gearing up for a speech though. "You know," she started, which is my cue to act like I'm paying attention, "we talked in my discussion group this morning about how none of us really takes our faith seriously."

"Really?" I thought this was an especially self-critical consensus for a group of ministers to arrive at, considering most ministers I know like to tell each other how great they are much more than engage in self-criticism.

"Well, if we say we're committed to serving the poor and living out the gospel, but we're not willing to sell everything we own and give it away, how well can our actions really match our words?"

"Hmm," I murmured, wondering where she was headed with all of this. I was sure there was a lesson for me to learn. There usually is. Here we are, sitting outside a homeless shelter, getting a minisermon from my preacher wife about materialism. Her angle was becoming clear.

"So," she sighed, "what was it you said you wanted?"

"Something cool," I said. "And something that you don't want."

"You're impossible."

"It's hard," I explained, "because most cool things I'd like, you'd like too. Maybe someone has invented a testicle warmer or something."

"I think you'd get tired of that."

"I'm pretty sure I wouldn't." About that time, her partners showed up and she ducked into the rain and ran toward the kitchen. I headed off to pick up Mattias at school, dreaming of enjoying my new testicle warmer while cruising around town on my new scooter.

* * *

Amy and I do a sort of debriefing before we fall asleep at night. Amy likes to pray, but I'm not really an out-loud kind of prayer, so our compromise is to share our best and worst experiences of the day. Amy's worst had to do with a guy she met at the shelter.

"He was a good looking guy," she said, with some surprise in her voice. "Tall, thin, nice tan. He had all his teeth still, which put him in the minority there. But his eyes were so sad. When he came through the food line, he thanked me more than once, but his eyes stayed fixed on my belly. I didn't get to talk with him any more than that, because he was so quiet, and went off by himself, but I get the feeling the thing he wants more than anything in the world is a family."

"And maybe a testicle warmer," I added. Amy ignored me.

"I wonder what happened," she said in a drowsy whisper, closing her eyes. We lay silently next to each other and drifted off to sleep, listening to the arrhythmic patterns of the rain dancing off the windows.

Lightning struck this young man's life. It would be convenient—and I'd suggest, highly judgmental—to enumerate the many reasons why this guy was where he was. Some of his situation likely was his own doing, but sometimes you just happen to be in the wrong place at the wrong time and lightning strikes. We try to give our kids lessons to help them avoid the biggest lightning rods, but this ensures nothing. He's somebody's son, no matter what's happened in his life.

At the root of compassion is, for me, seeing each person as someone else's child. Even that child-diddling priest was someone's boy once, spun from the same stuff as the rest of us. Maybe that's what's scariest about it, considering the prospect that each of us, our kids included, has in ourselves the capacity to become both victim and predator. And no matter how much damage we inflict, we still hold some potential to love and be loved.

I'm not saying it's in my nature to respond to such exploitive behavior with love, but I'd hope and pray that others would step up and do everything they could for my loved one if lightning were to strike.

CHAPTER 18

nesting instinct

Mom, please give me some space.

—Mattias, 3 years, 0 months

There's a phenomenon among women called nesting. It's the kind of behavior you see when you first move in with a chick and she starts rearranging all of your stuff. Most of what you owned before will either be put in the closet, stuffed in the corner, or shoved under the bed until it's given away, most likely while you're at work. Suddenly you look around and see no traces of yourself in your own home anymore.

That's nesting.

Many women have an irrepressible need to move things around, color coordinate, and basically get their own little feng shui going on. And most of the time, guys and their sense of place, fashion, utility, and personal value systems do not match with the nesting instinct.

This stuff goes very deep, biologically, too. Most women can't help it. The reason they're throwing out your neon beer sign is not because they think it's tacky, but because millions of years of evolution are warning her brain that it might attract predators. And she didn't throw away your favorite T-shirt because it stinks; it's because the pheromones from your highly masculine body might draw other women to your lair.

The net effect to you though is that you no longer have any say about your living environment. You are forever a guest in your own home, welcome to come and stay a while as long as you move nothing, put your clothes away, and basically don't leave a trail.

There are benefits to the nesting phenomenon too. Even those women who have never seen the shiny side of a stove suddenly get this desire to be prolifically domestic. Amy started making pies the other day so fast that I've hardly been able to eat them fast enough. This is from the woman who I've watched burn instant rice. And I'm not just being mean to say I think she could discover a way to scald water. But she went to this old lady's house from our church, learned how to make all these fruit pies from scratch, and hasn't stopped since. Consider me a happier—and significantly fatter—man for it.

If your wife begins to nest, the best thing to do—and frankly, the only sane option—is to get the hell out of the way. You never know what may happen, and rest assured something of yours will disappear forever, but if you leave the house you'll either come back to a clean house, a kitchen full of baked goods, or if you're not so lucky, a knitted pair of booties.

The whole baby thing puts the nesting instinct into hyperdrive. If you don't already have a room set aside for a nursery before your wife gets pregnant, that room will most likely end up being any workout room, music room, or other kind of sanctuary you have in the house. Plan to move all your favorite crap to the garage, if you're lucky, and get used to helping hang wallpaper borders, assembling baby furniture, and being asked which Pooh Bear mobile you think goes better with the Eeyore table lamp.

We already know which room is going to be the nursery, mostly because there's only one bedroom left. However, it's caused a chain reaction of problems we've yet to overcome. This whole dilemma about space started back when we decided to convert one of our bedrooms—which was Mattias's old nursery—into a master bathroom. I could see in my mind the issues that would arise if we ever decided to have another baby:

The old nursery would be gone, so the new nursery would have to go in the guest bedroom.

We can't be without a room for guests, so the only other place for the guest room furniture to go is up in the attic.

The attic is where my office is.

See the problem?

Now one of Amy's contentions is that I don't use the office that much, but one reason for that is that it gets so cold up there in the winter. In the summer, I could type naked and still risk passing out from heat exhaustion. We had someone helping us insulate the attic after we got a new roof, but he quit—guess why? It was too frigging hot up there!

If it's too hot for a roofer, what do you think it'll do to a pansy-ass writer like me? And no, I have not taken a day off to try to install the rest of the insulation myself. There are many reasons I became a writer and one of them is to avoid working hard.

The other thing that some women have a hard time understanding is that, for guys, having a space of our own is not so much about using it as it is about knowing it's there. It's easier for me to survive having twenty dinner guests in my house knowing that I have a little happy place waiting for me up in the attic. I even have a minirefrigerator up there, and even though it has nothing in it right now, it totally could hold a twelve-pack of beer or more. That's awesome.

So this little baby is threatening to displace me from my happy place. But what's the big deal? Babies are tiny and they'll sleep anywhere. I'd be happy to give up my sock drawer in order to keep my office intact. Or how about the bathtub? That kid could grow for years and still have plenty of room in there. Sure, I know what you're thinking; I'm so inhumane for suggesting my newborn baby sleep in a bathtub, but think back to the parties you used to go to when you were younger. Remember when you were hammered and the night was wearing on and you'd go in to take a leak? Remember how incredibly comfortable that bathtub looked and how all you wanted to do was curl up in there against the cool porcelain and take a nap?

It's also an awesome place to barf, which is perfect both for drunks and babies, both of whom do that plenty.

The other thing Amy's talking about is getting a nanny. Now the initial idea of a nanny is killer to any guy—have some young girl hang around your house and help take care of the kids in her thong bikini. But they're also expensive and some just can't pull off the T-back suit. So Amy's idea is to let the nanny live with us in the attic to help offset some of the costs.

On first blush this makes sense, but then I got to thinking about it. Why in the hell does she get my attic if I can't have it? I thought it was oh so important to keep that set aside for guests. And what if a dude ends up being the most qualified nanny? Do I really want some college guy living right over my bedroom?

No, I don't.

So there's a lot up in the air right now. I don't have any answers, or big revelations, or emotional hooks for this chapter either. I just needed to vent.

Maybe I'll go have some pie.

CHAPTER 19

same old sh*t

Me: *If you want to watch TV, you need to poop in the potty.*

Mattias: *I know, dad; you can poop in the potty, then you can watch TV, and I'll sit next to you.*

—Mattias, 2 years, 11 months

One of the coolest things about kids is that you see parts of yourself in them all the time.

That's also the worst thing about having kids, sometimes.

Some folks might say I'm picky about certain things, but I prefer to think of myself as discriminating. Along the same lines, while there are those who would label me as obsessive, I consider myself focused.

Focused discernment comes back to bite me in the ass quite often in the form of a blond-haired, blue-eyed future litigator who has, thus far, never been wrong in his entire short life.

I should back up and explain that my day today actually started yesterday in a sense, and even the night before that. It would be nice to have one of those supposed compartmentalized lives where work stays at work and home waits until you get home, but my line of work just doesn't lend itself to that. Usually, it's just all one big, messy ball of shit.

Amy had gotten up before me and my head was still cloudy from a lack of sleep and a beer or two more than I'm used to on a Tuesday night.

"Hey, I have to go soon," she said. "I have a meeting."

"More meetings, great," I mumbled, rifling through the paper and sipping my coffee.

"Mattias is still in bed," she hollered over the hair dryer.

"You sure?" I asked, a little rattled by a disturbing dream I'd had last night.

"What?"

"Forget it," I shrugged.

"Anyway, he will need breakfast and I haven't laid his clothes out."

"OK."

"And he didn't take a bath last night," she said, with a mouth full of toothpaste.

"Awesome."

"And also, he doesn't have a lunch yet. You'll need to make one for him."

"Seriously honey?" I sighed, "I just woke up and you're already piling all this on me. I've got a lot to do this morning too."

"I know," she said, "but I'm already late." Notice a trend in our lives?

She kissed me on the forehead and headed out the door, just as I heard the door to his room pop open. The first thing I did was give him a big, long squeeze to reassure myself that he really was there, all in one piece, and not splattered all over the walls of his room like he had been in my dream.

Then the circus started.

I got him the breakfast he asked for, but he didn't like the cereal after a few bites. He decided he wanted something else. I sprinkled some cinnamon sugar on what he had to try to doll it up, and he made it through a couple more spoonfuls and then decided it just was no good.

Instead of getting more cereal, I gave him a banana. He made it about halfway through and stopped. "It's too mushy in the middle," he said.

"So eat around it," I told him from upstairs, trying to pick through the basket of laundry for a halfway coordinated outfit, just to avoid Amy's inevitable comment later.

"I don't want it," he insisted. "I want yogurt Cheerios."

"You already got cereal."

"Yeah," he said, starting to whine, "but all the sugar went away."

"Sugar dissolves," I said, with an armful of clothes. "It doesn't go away. You just can't see it."

"What's 'dissolve' mean?"

"It means when something disappears but it's still there, kind of."

"So if you're invisible," he asked, "you dissolve?"

"If you're in milk," I said, "yeah, I guess so."

"Why would you be in milk?'

"I have no idea," my shoulders sagged. "You're going to be hungry if you don't eat more."

"I'm done," he said. "I don't want any more. Can I watch TV?"

"No," I said, laying his clothes out in the order he likes to put them on, "we have to get going. Daddy has a busy day."

"But I ate my breakfast."

"Not really."

"But I want to watch TV," he protested. For those reading who already have kids, the old "but I want to" mantra is chillingly familiar. It's the verbal equivalent of bamboo shoots under the fingernails.

"Well, I want a book deal and I want world peace, but I'm not holding my breath for either one. Get dressed."

"What's world peace?" he asked, standing naked in the middle of the living room.

"Nothing you need to worry about," I said, "forget it." While I waited for him to get his clothes on, I made the mistake of opening my laptop up to see how many e-mails I had waiting for me: sixty-five.

Crap monkeys. I'm going back to bed.

"I have to wash my hands," said Mattias. "They're sticky from the banana."

"Fine, go wash them," I said, glancing up over the top of my computer.

"But I want to use the sink in the kitchen."

"Go ahead."

"I'm too short."

"Then grow."

"Dad," he said, "that's mean. You need to pick me up so I can wash." I put the computer down and went in to hoist him up to the sink.

"There," I grunted, setting him back down. "Now go get dressed." I had a conference call coming in a little more than two hours and about twice as much work as I could get done between now and then to wade through to avoid making an ass of myself on the phone.

He had no sooner gotten around the corner into the living room before he came back around, still naked. "I have to wash my hands again," he said.

"Why?"

"Because I touched the red chair and it had hair on it, and now the hair is on my hands, and I can't get my clothes on with hair on my hands."

"Fine," I grumbled, "come here." We repeated the hand-washing ritual and I ushered him back into the living room just as I heard the chime on my computer indicate I had more e-mails coming in. Mattias picked up his Denver Nuggets jersey and almost had it over his head, when he stopped, set it down, and made a face.

"I have to wash again, dad."

"You're kidding me."

"Look," he thrust his hand under my nose, "there's more hair."

"Your mom just vacuumed yesterday," I said. "You must be a freaking hair magnet." We washed his hands a third time, and I practically drop-kicked him into the living room to get dressed while I made his lunch. He got as far as his socks before it all came to a grinding halt again.

"These socks are too small," he said. "I need different socks."

"They're not too small," I said, pouring a can of soup into a plastic travel bowl. "They're ankle socks. Your Uncle Matt wears them, so they're cool."

"Why does Uncle Matt wear ankle socks?" he sat in the middle of the kitchen floor, wrestling with the socks.

"I have no idea. Put it on your list to discuss with him next time you guys chat."

"I can't get these on," he threw them down on the floor. "I need help." I set the food on the counter and sat down with him to contend with the notorious ankle socks. They actually were pretty hard to get on.

"There," I said, stretching the second one over his heel, "now go finish getting dressed."

"I don't want shorts," he complained. "It's cold outside and I need jeans."

"It's a high of eighty-eight today," I said, grabbing a tube of string cheese. "You'll be fine."

"But those shorts are too big," he said. "They'll fall off when I run across the playground."

"We'll get you a belt."

"I need it now or I can't keep my shorts on." I stopped lunch preparations and ran upstairs to find a belt. It was buried underneath fourteen pairs of shoes that are too small for him to wear anymore. Why we still have them in his closet is a mystery to me. By the time I got downstairs, he had his shorts on—backward.

"You put your shorts on backward, buddy," I said.

"No I didn't."

"The button's back there by your butt," I said. "That's backward."

"I put them on right," he argued, "then they changed by magic."

"Fine," I sighed, laying the belt on the chair, "change them back."

"I need help with my belt."

I'm going to have a heart attack before this kid even gets to school. We get his shorts turned around and sufficiently secured to avoid a playground nightmare, and I leave him with only his shoes to go while I finish his lunch. He came in completely dressed, finally, and peered over the counter.

"What did you make me?"

"Soup, cheese, crackers, an apple, and lemonade."

"What kind of crackers?"

"Square ones."

"The kind with the lines like this?" he demonstrated some inscrutable pantomime with his finger, intended to outline some sort of design on some cracker he's seen at some point in his lifetime.

"I dunno, they're just freaking square."

"Let me see them," he insisted. I took them out of his *Backyardigans* lunch bag and let him inspect the design on the crackers. Thankfully, they passed. I zipped up the contents, which always is followed by Mattias inspecting the zipping job we've done to make sure that there's no daylight around the end of the zipper area.

We gave birth to Rain Man. Next thing you know, he'll be counting toothpicks on the floor and freaking out if it's two minutes until Judge Wapner is on.

Finally, with him fully dressed and with a lunch approved by the four-year-old FDA squad, we head out the door. We get out to the car and I realize his car seat is missing. "Shit," I said, peering over the back seat.

"That's a potty word, dad," said Mattias. "You're not supposed to say 'shit.' 'Shit' is a bad word, dad." He loves an excuse to correct me and have a legitimate excuse to use obscenities.

"Thank you, son," I rubbed my eyes with my fingers. "You wait here. I'm going to go look for your seat in the house." For some unknown reason, it was sitting in the living room, right next to the door by which I had just left the house. How in the hell did I miss that?

"Dad," came a voice from the trunk of the Xterra, "look what I found."

"God only knows," I lowered my head.

"It's your guitar stand."

"Sure is," I reached back to pull him up into the middle seat.

"Did you use this last night at the Monkey Bar?"

"Yep, I used it at the monkey bar." I fastened him in and shut his door but could hear his howls of protest before I could get around to my door on the other side.

"Dad," he said, with a look of great distress on his face, "this seatbelt is too loose."

"So tighten it."

"But it's all twisted, see?" he lifted the harness, hoping to convince me of his plight. I reached back, gave the belt a yank and tightened it up against his lap.

"There, you're fine."

"But it's still twisted," he argued.

"So am I," I scowled. "Deal with it."

I finally got back home with about an hour and a half left before my meeting, my list of e-mails had grown by about fifteen or so, but I just had to close it down and pretend it didn't exist. By some freak occurrence, I happened to pack several hours of work into that ninety-minute span and make my call without incident.

"So how's your day going, mister mom?" came a voice across the line from seven hundred miles away.

"Oh, pretty good so far," I sighed, picking up my notepad. "Same old, really."

Carrie Fisher did a monologue recently where she talks about how it is that she can stand in front of a group of people today and laugh with them about the pain from her past. She says it's all about location, location, location. In the moment, it sucks, but as time goes by, the sucky parts actually seem funny in the larger context of an entire life.

Here's to laughing about this, sometime in the distant future.

a glimpse of the worst

(Pointing to a motorcycle that passed by)

That was so loud, it hurt my food.

—Mattias, 2 years, 11 months

It was too hot by Colorado standards to do much of anything yesterday. We had gone to the fair earlier in the afternoon to hear a friend sing at the local artist stage, but by the time her set was done, I had a massive case of June Ass (the trickle of sweat trailing down into the crack of your butt) and Amy was getting groggy from the sun.

When we picked Mattias up from school, he wanted to know, like he always does, what we were going to do. Getting him to settle down inside after a day of school is no easy thing, but we tried plopping him in front of Spongebob for a while.

Hey, don't judge me. It was friggin' hot, OK?

He got restless in a half hour or so and we finally relented, letting him go out and ride his scooter up and down the sidewalk while we hid under the shade of the porch. The heat doesn't seem to bother him, sweat tricking down the bridge of his nose, his cheeks blossoming like a pair of cherry tomatoes. But he was happy, which means everyone's happy, so we let him keep going.

As I sifted through the afternoon mail, I heard a shrill noise on my right. I looked up just in time to see a cargo van hurtle down our one-way street the wrong way at about forty miles an hour and into the intersection, where there was a sedan already in his path. The driver of the van, a scrawny construction worker in his twenties with a scraggly goatee, was on his mobile phone and didn't even apply his brakes before he plowed into the fifty-something Hispanic woman driving the sedan, her teenage daughter in the passenger seat.

Though the woman tried to avoid him, his speed prevented her from doing any more than slamming on her brakes, which caused him to plow into her driver-side fender rather than her door, which would have been his target otherwise. Amy and Mattias looked up just after the van sent the sedan into a spin, finally coming to rest against the curb of the cross street, nearly facing the opposite direction she had originally been heading.

I jumped from the porch steps and Amy called to Mattias as we saw the van swerve out of control, veering at nearly full-speed toward our front yard. With little time to do more than embrace my son and watch helplessly as the scene played itself out, the driver finally compensated, sending the van up onto the curb and into a grassy bank opposite us.

He was never really that close to hitting us, but when several thousand pounds of metal comes flying out of control toward your kid, the images that pass through your mind are less than pleasant.

The police and ambulances arrived within minutes and I, as the only eyewitness who had seen the whole thing from beginning to end, recounted the scenario to a young cop with a notepad. Amy, who is fluent in Spanish, was speaking to the woman behind the wheel, who was both in shock and no small amount of pain. Her daughter was in tears, walking up and down the sidewalk, apparently looking for someone who wasn't there.

I know enough Spanish to gather that Amy was helping to reassure the woman, to ask her to stay in her seat, and to find out where she was in pain. They exchanged a few words until the woman came out of a cloud. "You know, I can speak English fine," she said.

"Right. English, OK," Amy said, herself somewhat rattled by the chaos. By now, neighbors were coming out of their homes and one of them went and sat next to Mattias, who was sitting on the curb, his plastic helmet still pressing down on top of his ears. We only learned later from Susan, our neighbor, about the conversation between him and her.

"Well, that was pretty exciting." She said to him.

"No, it wasn't," he shook his head. "It was loud and it made me jump." He paused for a minute and then continued. "And I'm upset that there aren't any adults with me to keep me safe."

"Well, that's kind of why I came over," explained Susan, "since your parents have to talk to the police right now."

Susan joked that not being included in the "adult" category, given her small stature, reminded her of a college roommate who once commented that she wasn't big enough to be a twenty-year-old. I guess she hasn't really grown since.

But the point I think Mattias was trying to make was that he was freaked out and wanted his parents. To him, we're adults, figures of permanence, security, and something to depend on. Now I could be reading much more into this than my ego deserves, but he wanted us to be there.

It was a sobering, and at the same time, strangely encouraging experience. On the one hand, the experience of seeing a giant cargo van careening toward your son is enough to put you off dinner. In fact, I skipped dinner after that. But it's also a little window into Mattias's world, one that, even at four years old, he doesn't offer liberally. He's a fiercely independent kid. If he had a motto, it would be "I can do it myself."

But when it comes down to the gritty moments, when we're looking for something to fall back on, it's nice to know he was looking for us. I'd love to credit my superlative parenting skills, but it's more likely attributable to basic biology. As Bono says on U2's song "One", we get to carry each other. Sure it's work, but it's also good to be needed sometimes.

x and y

*I'm going to go potty with my penis, but my cheetah
puppet can't go potty because he doesn't have a butt.*

—Mattias, 3 years, 1 month

I went into a fast food restaurant recently to pick up some fuel for
the road. Mattias usually eats pretty healthy food, but when we're
traveling he knows it's time to cash in, so he requested the kids' meal
with fried, pressed chicken parts. Hey, who am I to stand in the way of
a child's dream?

When I got to his meal in the order, the cashier asked me if it was
for a boy or a girl. *Kind of a personal question,* I thought to myself. *Since
when do they start screening you to make sure you're actually buying it
for a kid?*

"I know the toys in those meals are awesome and all," I said, "but
it's really for my kid. He's out in the car." I felt like a moron explaining
myself, but once I was committed it was hard to stop.

"No," she said, "they have different toys for boys and girls."
Seriously? Does the boy one have a part that requires a penis to operate
or something? I decided that my desire to take this totally pointless but
fascinating discussion any further was trumped by my family waiting for
me in the car and the growing line of hungry mountain townspeople
queuing up behind me.

They handed over a bag with the kids' meal in it, and out of
morbid curiosity I pulled the toy out. Sure enough, there was an action
figure, complete with a sword. No penis-triggered levers or buttons,
but an intimidatingly phallic weapon of war at least. Aside from being
brazenly violent, it was covered in ads for some new, equally violent,

113

summer movie. No wonder these meals are so friggin' cheap: they come sponsored by Disney. I tossed it in the trash on the way out.

Mattias was so blissed out on his nuggets that he didn't even notice the missing toy, which made for a much better drive home. I was kind of surprised he ate at all considering he'd just had three blueberry pancakes, some bacon, and a banana a few hours before, and a ham and cheese sandwich just as we got in the car. I thought he might just nibble at the food as an excuse to get a cheap plastic toy, but he devoured everything, ripped a satisfied burp, and promptly passed out, forehead folded limply over onto his knees.

The boy can eat.

The nature-versus-nurture debate is nothing new, but examples like this leave no doubt that commercial America does its share to mold my kid's gender identity. And to tell you the truth, I'm not too impressed with Corporate America's parenting skills. They pretty much suck, actually.

Who knows how much we as parents contribute to gender roles, even when we try not to? We resolved not to impose things on him like what toys are girl or boy toys, and what girls can or can't do versus boys. But I also recognize when I do things at a nearly unconscious level, like calling little boys "buddy" and little girls "sweetie." I'm sure I'm also more rough-and-tumble with Mattias when I play with him, partly because he's more aggressive and also because he's built like a three-and-a-half-foot-tall brickhouse. But how much of his aggressiveness comes from how I treat him, causing a sort of self-feeding cycle?

I'm more of the disciplinarian in our family, but would it be different with a girl? Even imagining having a little girl gives me distinctly different feelings than with a boy. Neither is better than the other, but they're not gender blind. Should they be? Can I even help parts of the ways I treat my kids? Is there some deep, evolutionary necessity even in the words I choose and the facial expressions I offer?

In other words, maybe it's not such a bad thing, treating boys and girls differently. Maybe it's the notion of gender blindness that is off base, fighting against an unstoppable force of nature that's actually there for a reason.

The reality is that we are different, and as Martha Stewart says, that's a good thing. Not everyone is on board with me on this, which is fine, but I'm a fan of how boy and girl parts fit together. I'm always amazed that women find us guys attractive, but I'm sure grateful that most do. In our relationship, we pride ourselves in being more egalitarian than the stereotypical father-knows-best family, which has its benefits and liabilities. I get jokes about being a pastor's wife, and I probably get more weirded-out about a second kid than dads who aren't as involved in home life. Amy has to try to balance aspirations for a career and the urge to be a mom. It's far from perfect, but it's a life nonetheless.

So how do you teach a boy to be a man in a world where the very idea of "man" is a moving target? And as far as a girl goes, I'd spoil the crap out of her, but I hardly know how to raise a woman-to-be in the twenty-first century. I can handle the basics for either sex I think, like teaching and modeling values for a life of kindness, generosity, and hopefully for leaving the world better off than we find it. But do you teach the gender identity stuff or does it take care of itself? And how much of the cultural messages do you let through and which ones do you fight against?

We go in later this week for the twenty-week ultrasound. That's the one where, if you want to, you can find out the sex usually. I say *usually* because part of it depends on the baby's position. If they're all folded up and hiding their junk, you may not be able to tell. They can also be wrong, but the better technology gets the more certain they are. We didn't find out with Mattias, which was fine. We did things pretty much the same regardless of whether he was going to be a girl or boy. It was also pretty cool because people had to go with gender-neutral colors, toys and everything. He's still a 110 percent boy, regardless of our efforts to be the parental equivalents of Switzerland on the subject. So much for nurture.

This time though, Amy really wants to know. We haven't talked a lot about it, but it's abundantly clear that part of the motivation behind her wanting another child was, more specifically, to have a girl. I reminded her that the only surefire way to go about it was to adopt, but the urge to procreate won out over the control over innies and outies. Now we're facing the result of that choice.

I'll admit that I'm a little bit nervous about finding out. I don't really mind either way, although I think it would be fun to have one of each. And although gender doesn't guarantee the sort of disposition the kid will have, most of the little girls I know are so much more laid-back than Mattias. That sounds awesome to me. But the main reason I'm anxious is because of Amy. With the severity of her postpartum issues last time, I'm on high alert about how the letdown of having a boy might affect her. Of course, I know she'd love the kid the same regardless, but there's this lingering expectation that's hanging there and the last thing I need is a prepartum or midpartum episode, or whatever a midpregnancy freak-out would be called.

We also have lots of people hanging on to their old baby clothes, waiting to hear which we're going to have. This is another example of gender expectations molding the baby's identity, even before it takes in its first breaths of air. It's not like making a boy wear pink will turn him into a serial killer, but folks will sure look at you cross-eyed. As much as we'd all like to think we're of independent minds, we all buckle to social pressures in one way or another.

Personally, I'm looking forward to not calling the kid "it" anymore. It's hard to bond with something before you can even tell what sex it is. That'll tell you something about how profoundly important gender identity really is to us. I'd like to say it doesn't matter but it does, obviously. I don't care if it's a boy or a girl, but there's a part of me that can't move forward with my own emotional connection until I know one way or the other. Call it superficial or a weakness of character, but this time I need all the help connecting with this kid that I can get.

*　*　*

Well, the uterus portraits were conclusive. It was a family affair, this ultrasound, with Mattias in tow and Amy's mom, Suzie, joining us as well. We were all crowded around the little monitor, trying to decipher the blobs shifting across the screen since Doctor Personality spoke as if he had already reached his verbal quotient for the day. And once we were told what we were looking at, there it was, plain as fetus genitals stuffed inside a womb and photographed with black-and-white sound wave images can be.

The first two thoughts that went through my mind as I began to recognize my kid's goodies on the screen were

1.   I am so screwed.
2.   How in the hell am I going to learn to clean a baby vagina?

"It's a girl," sighed the deadpan doctor, as if he was changing my wife's oil.

"How sure are you?" I asked.

"One-hundred percent." He nodded. That's when Amy lost it. Her relief and joy were, fortunately, way clearer than the pictures on the ultrasound. She would have come to terms with having a second boy, of course, but she wanted a girl more than anything and her happiness simply overflowed.

"Oh my God," she said, looking back at the screen, "there she is. Baby Zoe." Ahh, sweet relief. Baby "It" finally has a name. Let the pink frilliness begin.

We had promised Mattias that we'd go buy him some new shoes if he did well in the doctor's office, so we headed to the mall, which I knew would also lead us elsewhere. Within minutes, Amy and her mom were in the girly-girl sections of the baby clothes in the nearest department store they could find. We left with no less than a pink dress, several sweet pea gowns, and three pairs of white tights.

Mattias finally got his Lightning McQueen shoes, complete with blinky racing lights, and proceeded to demonstrate them and explain their function in exhaustive detail to every person who would indulge him long enough to allow him to launch into his monologue. "See these lights?" he'd say, stomping his feet firmly on the ground. "These go up along the sides here and they help you see me in the dark. They also make me look like I'm going really fast in the dark, but it's not dark here. It's OK, though. You can still see them. Watch," and off he went.

Suzie and Amy were giggling and fawning over the tiny clothes nearby, and I was still marveling at how I had just spent twenty-five bucks on some rubber shoes with LED lights embedded in them—with commercials for Disney across them, no less.

Try as I may, it seems that corporate America won out this time. Score one for you this time, you capitalist vermin, but we'll meet again come Christmas time, if not sooner. We'll see who has the last laugh.

If I were a betting man, I would put my money on the Suits.

good and evil

Mommy, if you cry, I will take you to the zoo and then to jail.

—Mattias, 2 years, 9 months

I've written about Mattias's change of schools this year already. We really liked the progressive sort of approach of his old school, but personnel and other administrative issues forced us to move on. The last thing I need, after all, is some Jerry Springer chair-smashing drama or the like in the middle of my kid's preschool room.

We looked into every option we could find. Because of his age, he's not allowed to enter kindergarten yet, even though he's reading, spelling, and doing basic math already. We also looked into other private prekindergarten options, and this was the only full-day program that had a solid program and didn't cost us a second mortgage and a testicle to do. The good part about him spending another year in preschool is that he has plenty to learn to keep up with other kids his age about taking turns, following directions, and basic social strategies. So it's not all bad that he's learning one letter a week still.

Mattias doesn't seem to mind either. We asked him the other day when he told us they were learning about the letter "P" all week if he had told his teacher he could read. "No," he shrugged, "I haven't really felt like it."

Fair enough. It's not like the kid has anything to prove, right? She'll figure it out soon enough.

The great news is that he loves his teacher, his friends, and his class. He has not complained once about going to school in the four months he's been there, which is a radical change from the days of daycare. But again, the downside is that the theology taught at this Missouri Synod

Lutheran School is not exactly in line with what we teach him at home or in our church. And as I said, though I'm not a fan of watering down Bible stories for Sunday school, I find it makes for some entertaining conversations.

"Dad," Mattias asked over dinner last night, "why did God flood the whole earth?" He was referring, of course, to the story of Noah in the Old Testament, which so many children's lessons revolve around, even if it is an apocalyptic display of carnage on a massive scale. But hey, it has cute animals in it, so that's cool.

This is when it would be really helpful to be a biblical literalist and just offer a pat answer. No such luck. I've learned not to rush my answers with Mattias, because I know from experience that if I offer him an off-the-cuff answer without thinking it through, he'll remember it until I'm ninety-seven and likely bring it up on my deathbed, challenging and questioning me into my grave.

"Your mom and I believe that this is a story about people trying to understand why bad things happen sometimes," I took a breath to stall and glanced at Amy, hoping she'd pick up the ball. She did, thankfully.

"Think about how long ago this story is talking about too," she said. "Nobody had maps of the whole earth, and most people didn't travel more than a hundred miles from home their whole lives. To them, the world was pretty small." I saw where she was going with this, and I liked it.

"Plus," I added, "most people had to live right by a river so they could have fresh water to drink, and for their animals and farms. So what do you think would happen to all of those people if it started raining really hard for a long time?"

"The rivers would go up?" he said. We benefit here from living between two pretty large rivers, so he's seen this firsthand.

"Right," said Amy, "and so if the whole area where they live flooded and all they can see in any direction is water, does it make sense they might think the whole planet was covered with water?"

"So it wasn't?" he asked, furrowing his brow. He usually does this when we say something that doesn't match up with his lessons from school.

"We don't really know," I said. "It could have been, but we think it's more likely that it was a big flood, but maybe not the whole world. After all, somebody had to be around to write the story down, right?"

"I guess so," he looked down at his plate of peas and carrots. "So why did God do that?"

"I don't know that God did, exactly," I said, showing my commie liberal theological roots. "Sometimes when bad things happen, we just try to figure out reasons why. Sometimes it's easy to blame it on God. I suppose God could flood the earth if he decided to, but that's not really the kind of God I believe in."

"Me either," said Amy.

"Maybe they just did something bad," he said. "So they thought God was mad at them."

"Makes sense to me," I said. "But my favorite part of the story isn't about how bad stuff happened, but how Noah did what God wanted him to do and that he took care of his family and lots of other animals on the earth."

"What about Adam and Eve?" He likes to change subjects without notice to keep us on our toes. "Why did God send them out of the Garden?"

"The story says they ate from the Tree of Knowledge," said Amy.

"What's that?" he asked.

"To me," I said, "the whole story is talking about how God made us how we are so we could make our own choices. God gave us everything we need on the earth to live a good life, but somehow we always find a way to get into trouble."

"Think about all the toys at home you have." Amy said. "You have a lot, right?" he nodded. "What if I told you that you could play with any toy you have except your Thomas trains? Which toy do you think you'd want to play with the most?"

"My trains," he said.

"Yeah, we're funny that way," I said. "We all do that kind of stuff. Now what if you had all these great toys and then you see a kid with another toy you really like. Do you think about all the ones you already have or the one you don't have?"

"I want the other kid's toy."

"Right," I nodded. "Well, the tree in the story is like the other kid's toy. You don't really need it, but there's something inside you that wants it just because you can't have it."

"Who is the snake?" he asked. This kid never gives up.

"I'm not so sure it was actually a talking snake," I said, trying to think of the simplest way to explain my take on biblical metaphor. "You know that voice in the back of your head when you see something you really want that just gets hooked on that thing and says 'I want it, I want it, I want it' over and over again?"

"Uh huh."

"Like when you see candy you want, or a toy."

"Yeah, I really want it, so my brain tells me I want it over and over."

"Right. So instead of making us just do the right thing all the time, we were made so we can choose to make good choices or bad ones. And the snake in that story, to me at least, is the voice that tries to make you do just what you want, no matter what is right for you or anybody else."

"So," he looked toward the ceiling as he processed, "if you choose to be good then you're good, and if you choose to be bad then you're bad."

"Exactly."

"And the snake is the voice in my head that tells me to make bad choices?" I looked at Amy and smiled.

"Send this kid straight to seminary," I said, sitting back in my chair with a sigh of relief.

We talked a little more about grace and the nature of forgiveness, greed, and what this and that story was about in the Bible. It's truly a miraculous experience in itself to witness a young, fresh, and uncluttered mind take in these ideas, mold them to his particular reality, and then carry them around as part of his worldview.

My hope is that he'll get the chance to share these stories with Zoe some day, to ask her what she thinks they mean, and to give her his own understanding of God. Someday, in many unexpected ways most likely, his understanding of things such as the Bible, God, faith, religion and so on will diverge from mine. But that's the way it should be.

For now, I'm lucky enough to be the one he comes to, along with Amy, to ask such incredible questions. If kids usually tend to turn into what their parents resist most, ours may likely become raging fundamentalists that embrace the kinds of things Amy and I work hard to undo. We can't make the choices for them, but we can at least give them a chance to see things another way.

But I'm drawing the line at felt boards. If they become fundies, the least they can do is be more original about it. I think they owe us that much.

CHAPTER 23

beginnings and endings

*Hey everybody! I can ride my bike with two wheels and
not fall down for a long time! Yay me!*

—Mattias, 4 years, 10 months

I had a dream a couple days ago, the night before my thirty-seventh
birthday. I dreamed that I died, which I thought was impossible to do
but I was still hanging around earth as a ghost, even though no one
could see or hear me. It was kind of like Patrick Swayze in that cheesy
90s movie, but with me as the schmaltzy actor in the lead.

It was incredibly frustrating trying to get Amy's attention, to let her
know I was *right there*, even as she cried and moped around the house in
my apparent absence. After a while, I got pretty pissed off about the whole
situation, trying to figure out why it was that I'd be forced to linger in such
a state where it seemed like there was nothing I could do, except wait
around for Whoopie Goldberg to show up and interpret for me.

Then I figured it out. In the dream, Amy was still six months
pregnant, like she is now, and the idea was that if anything happened
to Zoe before she was born, she would need a kind of guide to help
her over to the other side. So I was there to act as some sort of spiritual
crossing guard in case my unborn child didn't make it to full term.

Lovely dream, right?

I woke up pretty rattled by the emotional effects of the dream and
also to the reality of being a year older. My kid hammered out a fairly
recognizable version of "happy birthday" on his keyboard, and after a
kiss from my wife and a couple of cups of coffee, most of the fallout
from the night before had faded.

Amy's coming to the end of her second trimester, which for those
of you who have not experienced it firsthand means she's moving out

of the "this pregnancy thing isn't so bad after all" phase, and into the "get this thing out of me before my uterus falls out on its own" phase. The latter period will last, for better or worse, for the next three months.

Aside from her transformation, Mattias is going through a lot of rather incredible changes lately too. He has been interested in learning how to ride his bike without the training wheels for a little while, and I haven't pushed it, but figured when he was ready he'd let me know. Last week that day came and I got the wrench out. I explained to him, as I pulled the little plastic wheels from the bike frame, that once they came off they weren't going back on. He understood, so we proceeded with the surgery.

It took all of about thirty seconds and one good fall to the pavement to get him screaming at me to put the training wheels back on. I learned, in the midst of one of his more colorful four-year-old tirades, that I had somehow caused him to fall and that he, in fact, had not authorized the removal of the wheels at all. I was a heathenous bastard, in so many words, for submitting my poor, innocent child to such degrading torture and I ought to commence with my prostrations, apologies, and amends posthaste.

Once he got all of that out of his system, including tossing himself to the sidewalk, arms and legs flailing in such a stereotypical fit that I took away points for being too derivative, he pulled it together. Without my help or persuasion, he pulled the bike back up, rolled it back up to the top of the slight hill in front of our house, and announced he was ready to try again.

Within ten minutes, he was running the length of the yard on his own and by the next day he was starting, stopping and cruising for ten minutes or so at a time with no help from either of us. It was a complicated experience, since on the one hand, I was incredibly proud of his bravery and persistence. But on the other, this little voice inside of me said, *damn, there goes my little baby.*

I know, only chicks are supposed to think things like that, but I'm putting it out there. I'm not ashamed. Not entirely, anyway.

A few days later, we were watching a football game Sunday afternoon, and Mattias said, "Dad, what's an alley?" I was only half awake, as I often am on Sundays after church, and I barely got my eyes open in time to see the tail end of a commercial on TV for some new American ale.

"You mean that?" I said, pointing to the last three letters.

"Yeah."

"That says 'ale,' buddy. It's a kind of beer."

"Oh," he shrugged, and went back to coloring the cover of one of my magazines.

About a year ago, when he has first started showing a lot of interest in letters and sounds, I bought him a collection of beginning reader books, called Bob Books. As is the case with many overly ambitious parents, I was jumping the gun by a lot, but when he started cherry-picking words from commercials, I figured it was time to pull out the Bob Books again.

At first, it was kind of like with the bike. Mattias had no interest in trying something new on his own, and frankly I was a tool for even suggesting such a thing. So I just brought the box of books along with us in the car on a trip recently, and by the time we got thirty minutes out of town, he had read all ten books in the collection out loud and was asking for more.

It's an amazing and humbling breakthrough moment when your kid learns to do things like ride a bike and read. There's hardly any other sense of joy, pride, and accomplishment that can compare. However, there's also this sense of planned obsolescence. You start to realize that the more you teach your children, the less they will need you.

Looking at things this way gives you an inevitable sense of the beginning of the end. It reminds me of a writer named Henri Nouwen who once said that every joyful moment is tinged with sorrow and that every new life is born into a cradle of death.

Not exactly the kind of guy you want preaching at your baby dedication.

His point, though obsessively morbid, is well taken. Think back to any happy occasion in your life. There's usually some sort of subtle—or not so subtle—undercurrent of melancholy. I had a minor breakdown when I was young around nearly every birthday, as I became aware of my mortality well before a typical midlife crisis.

Every day that passes is one less you have left to share with your loved ones. It's a dark way of looking at life, but without recognizing this shadow side of reality, it seems to me like the joyful times are somehow diminished. I know, this sounds like such a typically maudlin writer, decrying the turmoil of his perfectly comfortable life; call it a curse of being hyperobservant.

The good news is that once we accept, and even embrace, the idea that every good thing comes to an end, it's easier to stop worrying so damn much and spend more energy on enjoying the moment we're in. Looking back on the sense of sadness I had around Mattias's learning to ride a bike on his own, I thought instead about how amazing it was to be there when he finally made the breakthrough to independence.

Instead of thinking about how his learning to read means fewer times he'll crawl up into my lap and ask me to tell him a story, I focused on being thankful for his incredible mind and for being a witness to his miraculous development every day we have together.

As for the dream and my thirty-seventh birthday, they're pretty clearly related. After all, what the hell am I doing still making kids while I'm creeping up on forty? I'm going to be farting dust before Mattias and Zoe are out of college, if they go to college, and hopefully they'll stop asking me for an allowance before I start collecting retirement.

Sure, if things go the way they should, my ending will come before theirs and they will have other endings and beginnings both with and without me. Soon, this rollercoaster of a pregnancy will be over and Amy will be done being pregnant forever—barring some unraveled fallopian tube or a superhuman sperm that can leap tall vasectomies in a single bound.

It's weird to think of those kinds of things in our lives knowing they'll probably never happen again, but without their passing we'd never have the new beginnings that inevitably follow. In most cases, the ends are worth the beginnings they birth and even when they're not, another beginning is sure to be pretty close behind.

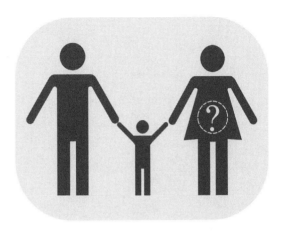

My Third Trimester

male bonding

Me: *Mattias, you're a pretty cool kid.*

Mattias: *Yeah, well, some men are made that way.*

—Mattias, 6 years, 5 months

I'm officially in love with an ear of corn. Baby Zoe is only about fourteen inches long, and weighs two pounds at best, but her power over my life is immeasurable. Sure, I've been warming up to the idea of having a daughter for months now, but the other day we got the chance to see her up close and personal.

A new clinic opened in town where they do what's called 4-D ultrasound, which is basically three-dimensional real-time video of your kid rolling around in the uterus. Not only could we see enough features of her face to recognize who she looks like, but we watched her smile, open and close her mouth, suck her thumb, and even grab her feet and lift them over her head, unladylike as it may be.

We also confirmed, even for my unscientific eye, that she is without question a girl. "There are her girl parts," said the technician, scanning her goods across the flat screen TV.

At first, I was a little concerned because her face—especially her nose—was all mashed flat, like someone had taped it down to her skull. But the tech explained it was a distortion of the imaging system, combined with being squashed in a small space, rather than some freakishly wide nose that would consume half her face. So that's good news.

What struck me at first was how much like Mattias she looks. I mean, before, I had these imaginary pictures in my mind of how she might look, with pigtails, riding her bike or kicking some middle school boy in the nuts for groping her. But now I *know* what she looks like and it's powerful. She's infinitely more real all of a sudden and I can't not love her.

It could be that Mattias senses the attention already being afforded the new little one or it could be something much less self-serving, but he has been incredibly affectionate lately, especially toward me. He makes things for his mom all the time at school, but in church recently they learned about writing love letters, which is based on a scripture by Paul. So he wrote his to me.

"This is for you dad," he said, beaming. He handed me a piece of folded construction paper with a stick figure on the front next to a ball and another straight line. "That's you with your mandolin," he said. "Look inside. I put all the things you like in there."

Fortunately he was ready to translate, as I did not immediately zero in on what exactly it was that I liked so much. "See," he said, "there's a monster with five eyes." I do love me some five-eyed monsters, I must admit. "There's an ice cream cone," he continued, "and some shapes." Gotta like the shapes. I'm a fan of shapes.

"What's this, buddy?" I asked, pointing to a circle with some lines drawn through it in an "X" pattern.

"It's a circle with some lines through it, dad," he said, exasperated.

"Wow," I squeezed him tight, "what an awesome card. I love it."

"I love you, dad," he closed his eyes and squeezed back. A parent never, ever hears that too much.

I was winterizing the house the other day and Mattias decided he wanted to help me. Though he's at an age now where he can focus long enough to engage in some basic household tasks, it still ends up taking two to three times as long to do anything with his "help" than it does to go it alone. But he has to learn and I do get some strange sort of manly ego boost from having my kid follow me around, helping me do man stuff.

"Why do we have to unhook the hoses from the house?" he asked.

"Because if the water freezes and they're still connected," I said, "they break the pipes inside."

"How?"

"Well, the water gets bigger when it freezes and it cracks the pipes."

"Can I do it?"

"Sure," I said, taking a few steps back. "Give it a try." I make a real effort to let him try things by himself at first, unless he asks for help. First of all, I've learned that he can do a hell of a lot more than I think he can, like riding his own bike now, dressing and bathing himself, and even doing some basic chores, so I'm more content now to let him discover his own limits rather than making assumptions.

This, however, was not one of those empowering moments. "It's too hard," he grunted. "I need help." I don't know about moms, but dads don't get tired of hearing that from their little guys either. Makes you feel necessary. We got the hose disconnected then moved on to our other tasks, each of which elicited at least another dozen or so questions.

I also recently went on a short trip out of town, which I'll talk more about in the next chapter, but when I got home after less than two days away, you'd have thought he hadn't seen me for a month. He ran to me, threw his arms around me and nearly knocked me over in the middle of the kitchen floor. It was tricky, balancing on my toes in a crouched position, hanging on to him with one arm and managing my bags in the other, but I wasn't going to be the first to let go.

I've also felt closer to Mattias, even when we're not physically together. He's been sharing more with me about his days, and I also am beginning to see more fruits of the lessons I've tried to impart to him, both in my own words and actions. One of the most reviled phrases of my childhood, often uttered by my dad, was, "do as I say, not as I do." Though I didn't know the term "double standard" back then, I knew that justified disparities between a parent's action and their moral lessons were based on crap logic. So I resolved to try to be as consistent with both as I could.

One example of this came the other day after Mattias spent some time with a buddy of his at the park. It actually was a boy he had just met while enjoying one of the final days of a Colorado Indian summer in the park, but for Mattias a couple of minutes and a willingness to be bossed around are the only needed criteria for lifelong companionship. The two went off and played while Amy talked baby stuff with the boy's mother. I actually wasn't there since I was working at one of the many jobs I've taken on in preparation for added baby expenses. So like many stories, I heard this one secondhand.

The boys came running back from the gravel around the "big boy" swings with a look of moderate dismay on their faces. When asked what was the matter, the other little boy looked up shamelessly and said, "That adult over there with the kids told us we were stupid."

"Are you sure?" Amy asked, not readily willing to believe that too many adults engage in unsolicited verbal assaults on four- and five-year-old kids.

"Yes, he did," said Mattias. "He called us stupid."

"So I told him and his friend they were f***ers," said the friend, matter-of-factly. There seemed to be not one ounce of shame in the retelling either. The moms explained his response, though impeccably timed, was not entirely appropriate. Later in the car, Mattias recounted all but the juiciest details of the story, which had been recounted by Amy, causing me to nearly choke on my coffee.

"Dad," he said, taking my hand, "that man called us names, and the boy called him a name back."

"It's sad when people are mean to each other with words, isn't it?" I said, smiling only on the inside.

"Yes, and I didn't say anything mean."

"That's good."

"I just said, 'Hey, you be nice.'"

"Yeah," I sighed, "but you can't really make people be kind if they choose not to be."

"But he was a meanie," he explained. "I just told him to be nice."

"I hear you, buddy. But I think he probably is old enough to know better. Being mean for him is just a choice, just like being kind can be a choice for you, even when other people decide to be mean."

"Yeah," he looked at his feet, sticking straight out ahead of him over the edge of the seat. "I should just turn and walk away."

Lesson learned. We held hands in the back seat of the car, watching the sunset bleed across the western mountain range together. I was so filled with love for him, for his mom, and for the baby yet to come that words could not have communicated it. Fortunately, the peaceful silence was testament enough to the togetherness we all felt, speeding down the highway together.

And for the record, that other kid had it right. Anybody who calls my kid stupid is a f***er, no question. I could not agree more.

big shift

Dad, I want to go with you to the meeting. You can play movies on the computer and when you say it's time to go, I won't even argue.

—Mattias, 5 years

The Piatt household is changing. For a while, Amy's nesting frenzy was contained within the baking sector, but it has effectively bled over into every other part of our lives.

It was determined by the maternal powers that be that it was time to get the nursery ready. Simple enough, right? Slap a crib in the corner of the guest room, put up a changing table, make room for a place to put crappy diapers, and you're done.

Or not.

It turns out that a baby needs a lot more room to sleep than I thought; in fact, it takes a whole frigging room. So basically, since we only had four bedrooms upstairs, one of which is now our master bath, the guest room is being converted into a nursery.

The thing is that guests still have to sleep somewhere. Personally, I think if you come to visit people with a new baby and a five-year-old, you should be happy to get any sleep at all, let alone get an actual room with an actual bed. But Amy's a little more hospitable than I am. The only option then is the attic, where my office/lair is.

This plan has started a sort of Mad Hatter's tea party shuffle in our house. We had been putting off fixing up the attic since it's just my office and I can either deal with it or work from the coffee shop. But guests and their delicate constitutions certainly can't be expected to undergo the same discomforts that the actual residents of the house have dealt with for years, so we resolved to fix it.

I should have seen the chain reaction that followed coming. We hired some guys to handle the insulation, because I have neither the time nor the motivation to spend my brief down periods lugging fiberglass up and down the stairs. So a couple of handymen took it on for us, which was great.

The thing is, we had also been talking for a long time about getting the springs on the garage doors fixed, and with these guys here, it seemed to make sense to have them do that too. No big deal, I figured, and I headed off to work in the mountains. When I get home though, the whole garage has been cleared out, swept clean and there's a dumpster the size of our living room in the driveway with piles of crap I didn't even know we had in it.

"No sense in fixing the garage if it's all filled with stuff," said Amy, which again made sense. "Took a little longer to get the garage stuff done this way, though."

"Like, how long?"

"All day," she said. "Two guys."

"And what about the dumpster?"

"Two hundred thirty bucks to unload it at the dump," said Amy, "so we might as well fill it up with anything we have been wanting to get rid of."

From there we sorted and tossed all the garbage we had been holing up in the attic, the basement, the back porch, and in all the bedrooms. That, combined with the old insulation, filled about half of the space inside the trailer of an 18-wheeler. It made me feel both like a pathetic slob and freshly rejuvenated, all at the same time. So we moved some of the stuff in the attic out to the new space in the garage so we could make room for the guest room furniture—oh, and there was no lighting in the attic, so we had to install that too—then we moved all the guest room stuff up to the attic, and then all the new baby stuff into the guest room.

Well, not quite yet.

First, of course, you have to eradicate any sign that it ever was anything other than a guest room. While the guys are around doing other jobs, why not have them retexture the walls, paint, and install a new ceiling fan? There was some study done that found the incidence of SIDS, which I still don't know what the hell it is, can be reduced by 50 percent or something, just by having better air circulation in the baby's room. I thought a box fan would be perfect in the window, but Amy didn't feel the same way about it.

I probably didn't mention that when the previous owners built an addition on the back, they decided it wasn't really important to insulate underneath where the entire thing was exposed to outside air from three sides and underneath. The pipes under this addition have frozen every single year since we moved in, and although I will really miss crawling under the house in the middle of the night, usually in subfreezing temperatures to solder exploded pipes, Amy convinced me that having them insulate there while they had the blower available made good sense.

Three grand and a couple weeks later, I called a stop to the remodel activities. There were plenty of to-do's on the list that didn't get any attention, but we're to a point where either all work stops or we're going to have to put baby Zoe on the black market to pay for all future home improvements, which kind of defeats the point really. Plus I don't even know what babies fetch on the open market these days anyway. Might not even cover it all.

The other shift is based around Amy's snoring. I should preface this by saying she usually sleeps as elegantly as a princess, but when pregnant, women's sinuses swell up because of the increased blood volume in their bodies. This causes, among other things, horrendous snoring. Other side benefits include swollen ankles, panting following trips up and down stairs, and probably some other things I've yet to attribute to blood volume. I've mentioned in earlier chapters her propensity for snoring during pregnancy, but it's gotten to the point that I've had to move to the bed in the attic. It's either that or reup my Xanax prescription, and I'd rather not medicate myself for the final few months of her gestation.

Good thing for me that we got the insulation done up there after all, I guess. Even though I'm booted from my normal sleeping spot, at least I'm not freezing my nuts off while doing it.

The third—and perhaps most significant—shift is an emotional one. The first trimester was marked by some nausea and mood swings, but Amy could still get around like normal, at least. The second trimester is the honeymoon phase when she, like most women, felt like Mother Nature herself, exhibiting the telltale "pregnancy glow."

Well that glow distills itself into a slowly smoldering animosity toward all male body parts in the home stretch. I, or more specifically, my sperm, did this to her. And they should be punished. To her credit, Amy usually catches herself and puts her bile into a hormonal and situational context before severing my head entirely, but there's also some good fun to be had in lopping it clean off, just for the sake of sport now and again.

I can't blame her. If she had been somehow responsible for my own stabbing back pain, cramps, ill-fitting clothes, erratic sleep patterns, and voraciously unpredictable cravings, I'd be pissed too. But remember—she told me to do it.

Mattias has decided to engage in a little shift of his own lately, in preparation for the new arrival. Twice in recent weeks, he's had accidents in his shorts, including once at school, prompting a spontaneous miniconference with his teacher. He's also been more emotionally fragile than Britney Spears after a good head shaving, tossing himself on the ground in abject fits of despair with no real warning or justification, at least from what I can tell. Obviously, he's doing some acting out to test the limits of a few things, like whether or not his parents will still love him, whether or not he's a baby anymore, and so on. Knowing this makes at a little bit easier to deal with. Sort of.

All of this probably would be manageable, actually, if it wasn't being compounded by the rest of the world's problems. In the course of one week, we had four people from church in the hospital at the same time, plus one other founding member in critical condition. Amy spent so much time in and out of emergency rooms that she actually started to develop a taste for soup in a Styrofoam cup. I'll give her credit for being available to help so many other people while dealing with her own stuff, although that usually means she's at the end of her emotional rope by the time we get back together in the evenings.

Guys, if you haven't figured out by now, part of your job during pregnancy is to be an emotional shock absorber for your spouse. That, and you're supposed to buy her whatever foods she requests any time of day or night, without question. Follow those two rules and you may survive pregnancy.

The four people who went into the hospital were all released within a few days, which allowed things to go back to almost normal for a couple of days. But things didn't turn out as well for Harry, the foundational member who was in the ICU.

It was sort of poetic that Amy and I planned his service, since the first thing he said to Amy after visiting Milagro for the very first time was "You can preach at my funeral." I guess he knew something we didn't.

We've sung together at funerals before as hired help, and we were both involved in her uncle's funeral, which took place only a couple of weeks after we moved to Pueblo. But this was the first church member we've buried.

Harry lived the very definition of a hard life. He entered the military at age seventeen, just toward the end of World War II, followed by three-and-a-half decades of backbreaking work in steel mills. By the time we met him he was stooped and hobbled by pain, but he never let his own discomfort compromise his attitude. Instead of being justifiably bitter, he resorted to the kind of mischief that only old people and little kids can get away with. He would chase Mattias around with the butt of his cane and tease guests about being in the wrong seats. At the end of every service, during the time of shared community prayers, he generally had some smart-ass quip to offer instead.

I'll give the guy credit for tenacity too. After they removed all his breathing tubes, Harry flatlined no less than eight times over the course of twelve hours, triggering many rounds of anticipatory family prayers and send-off songs. He finally waited until nearly everyone had left to die more or less alone, in the early hours of the morning.

Harry also had a way of getting the last word in too, and he was not about to let his memorial service go by without getting a final poke in. Before the actual memorial, there was an outdoor service just for the family where his ashes were scattered in the garden of a nearby graveyard. It was a cool, blustery morning, but the family asked me to play instrumental music during the scattering of ashes, following Amy's brief homily.

Trying to stay clear of the family, I stood far to the side and just as the first handful of ashes fell to the ground, a burst of wind carried a few stray ashes upward and right into my face.

You might not know it, but human remains can put a serious hurt on a guy's eyeball. It was like someone put their cigarette out on my eye, and it started watering like crazy. The good news is that my tears fit right in, making me look that much more empathetic. But in reality, I was just trying to be able to see.

"I think I got some Harry in my eye," I told Amy when we got back to the car. "Ornery bastard."

Looking around that circle of loved ones, at least before I got Harry in my eye, helped me realize what I have to look forward to, at least if I'm lucky. I know that sounds kind of morbid, and it's not like I'm building a life based on how many people will be at my funeral, but this man lived a very simple life: unremarkable by the world's standards. But for his wife of fifty-six years and his children, including an adopted daughter and a passel of grandchildren, he was a rock. He was their anchor.

So Harry made his last, big shift and we were fortunate enough to be there to see him off. If anything will put life's troubles, unpredictability, and hardship in perspective, it's death. It's all these shifts that ultimately make up a life, uncomfortable as they may be in the moment. I think the difference between viewing life as a chain reaction of crises strung together or as a worthwhile journey that ultimately derives positivity from the volatility is more or less a matter of choice; for the most part, we control our way of perceiving the world. You'll survive the fits. You'll get past the drama, but really it's not to be avoided; it's life.

Thanks for getting in the last word, Harry. I guess I can say with total confidence that I'll always carry a little bit of you with me. You may be permanently lodged in my tear duct, but you're there.

CHAPTER 26

intervention

> *Everybody in the world has a rectum, but God doesn't, because he's invisible.*
>
> —Mattias, 4 years, 11 months

We've all heard the cliché that's tossed around all too casually to kids about how they can be anything they want to be if they just try hard enough.

It sounds great, but in reality, it's crap. A kid may get it in his mind that he wants to be a pilot, but if his vision sucks, or if he's too short, or if he's epileptic, his chances of being a pilot are dim. There has been this movement in America to focus on building up kids' self-esteem, but this nurturing mentality has gone over a cliff and we've begun coddling our kids to the point that we're raising a generation of miniature narcissists.

If there's any doubt about the veracity of this, just look at the research. In a recent poll of school-age children who were asked what they wanted to be when they grow up, the number one answer was "famous." More than anything else in the world, our children now want to be adored for the rest of their lives.

Isn't that sweet?

Far be it from me to criticize our culture that celebrates such unfettered egotism. The real problem is that our kids have come to buy the line of crap we've sold them—that they're actually at the center of the universe.

Yeah, our kids are special, just like everybody else.

Our kids don't have to be rocket scientists or brain surgeons to be good people. And also, by focusing on "being something" way out in the future, it actually devalues what they are right now, which is amazing little human beings, capable of bringing joy, pain, wonder, humor, tragedy, and everything in between into the world, not tomorrow but today.

Instead of telling Mattias he can be anything he wants, I've started telling him he can be a whole lot of things and it will be up to him to decide that. But more important than what he may or may not be as an adult is what kind of person he is as a child. I want him to know he's basically a good person, and I also want him to know when he hurts people, when he makes bad choices, when he does things I can't do, and when things are entirely up to him to deal with, no matter how many hugs or encouraging words I offer.

I'm hardly the perfect parent, but I'd like to think that my obsessive observation of human behavior has taught me a few things. First off, to the Baby Boomers, I love you guys but you screwed up a lot of kids. All the divorces, consumption-driven lifestyles, and career fetishes didn't come without a cost. There's a ripple effect that will be felt throughout society for generations, global warming and pandemic credit addiction being a couple of prime examples.

But as for us twenty- and thirtysomethings, there's a saying from Twelve-Step programs that goes, "a hundred and eighty degrees from sick is still sick." Basically this just means that if you observe messed up behavior and endeavor to do just the opposite, you're no more than a reaction to all the bad things you're trying to avoid. So although we may be more available to our kids than our parents were, some of us are actually overparenting.

It's hard to hear, but it's not such a bad thing for your kids to get hurt, disappointed, screwed over, disillusioned, and the like early in life. Our job as parents is not to ensure that our children avoid pain, but rather to help them avoid unnecessary suffering and to give them the tools to deal with real-world problems as they will inevitably arise.

I understand where this overdone parental involvement comes from in some ways though. There's no better place to see the by-products of broken families and lives than in church. After only being involved in ministry now for less than ten years, I can see how some faith leaders can lose their sense of God; sometimes, all you see is so much pain, brokenness, and hopelessness that it's easy to start buying into the misconception that that's actually all there really is in the world.

But I know better.

I have a close friend, who we'll call Randall, who I've known since college. He's smart, funny, much more outgoing than I, and he was well connected enough to get me in all the local bars even though I was two years shy of twenty-one at the time. He broadened my social circles and between him and the guitar player in my college band, my mind expanded a bit too with respect to all things chemical.

Looking back, these were some of the best times of my young life. The problem is that it's hard when you're playing as hard as we did to notice when someone is doing more than just experimenting: when they're really dealing with a beast they cannot tame and with pain they cannot drink away. It turns out that this was the case with Randall.

I had tried before to help him out but nothing ever took. I confronted him about how much he seemed to drink and he'd shrug it off. Once I invited him to church with us and he absolutely flipped, he enjoyed it so much. Randall was the kind of guy who would dismiss religion in one breath and then engage me in hours-long conversations about God in the next. I knew there was a craving in him for something and I thought it couldn't hurt to see if, just maybe, that hole he was trying to fill was God shaped.

Randall was so excited after going to a service with us but when his mother, a lifelong conservative in every sense, learned what we were about, she told him he was better off not going to church at all than he was going to a place like that.

So that was the end of his experience with our commie church.

A couple of years ago, after he had sought counsel from me about a particularly difficult relationship, I sent him a letter laying out my concerns in stark terms. Basically I told him, in the most loving way I could, that he either had to stop drinking or he would die. For a week or more I heard nothing, which I took as the beginning of the end, but then one day he answered.

First, he thanked me for my concern and then he acknowledged that he most likely did drink too much. But he was pretty confident he had things under control and that he could quit any time. Now anyone who had had an addict in their family knows this line well. It's like they hand out a script among all habitual drinkers and say, "When your loved ones come to you some day and try to get you to stop drinking, say this."

What I didn't know was that he had shared the letter I sent him with his sister, the only member of his family with whom he is close. His dad died when we were in college and his mom and other sister are generally checked out, but his younger sister, who we'll call Sarah, has been through her own version of hell and thankfully has come out on the other side. So if anyone knew what he was going through, it was her.

I got the e-mail to call her a couple weeks ago, like I said, and when I reached her she explained that Randall was about to lose his job. She felt like it was time for an intervention, and she needed help.

Fortunately Amy's dad has been in recovery for more than two decades, and he has performed more interventions than I can count.

The next thing you know, he and I are on a last-minute flight to Texas to save the world, or at least to try to help Randall get into treatment. For those unfamiliar with how interventions work, you basically gather a group of the person's closest friends and loved ones, and each person reads a letter about how the substance abuse has compromised things in their lives or their relationship together. The subject of the intervention does not know what's going on until they get there, and by then a bag is packed for them and a four-week stay at a treatment center is generally booked and ready for them that day.

It's an emotional thing, being a part of just a critical life-or-death decision like that for someone you care about. You know how in the previous chapter I talked about crying on a four-year cycle or so? Well, I guess I had saved up, because the water works came on when I read my letter, then they went gangbusters when he agreed to accept help.

I realized later that there was a lot more going on underneath my own skin than relief that Randall was getting help. At the same time, I was mourning the relationship with my dad, particularly given that the break between us revolved around alcohol in some ways too. It was made all the more salient by the conspicuous absence of Randall's older sister and mom, who opted not to participate in the intervention.

How in the hell does that happen? How does a parent or sibling stand by and not do everything in their power to rescue their loved one from suffering and perhaps death? Then again, how does a grandparent miss out on years of his only grandson's young life and on the birth of his only granddaughter? How do families that were bound by blood drift—or break—apart? How can love turn so bitter?

All of this came welling up when Randall said two simple words: "I'm ready."

I recognize that I have no small amount of residual anger, both toward my dad for not being around and toward Randall's family for not being there. They live in the same city. There are flawed relationships everywhere you look, but that kind of lapse is in a whole different category.

Coming to terms with all of this bitterness, relief, fear, and other stuff all balled up together, all I wanted to do was get home as quickly as possible, hold my family tight, and never let go. But like I said before, the opposite of sick is still sick, and trying to build an illusion of shelter around your wife and kids is largely a waste of time. Sure, you can reduce certain risks, but I can't guarantee Mattias won't end up a junkie and I can't promise that I'll keep Zoe off the brass dance pole, though I'll do my damndest. I can't ensure forever and always that Amy will stick by me, any more than I could guarantee my dad would resolve that being a part of one another's lives is more important than personal conflict.

You can bury your head in the dirt and try to pretend like bad stuff will never happen, or you can fool yourself into thinking you have more agency than you really do over the outcomes, but neither reflects reality. You can guide, mold, and nurture, but never control. You can tip the odds, but never get a guarantee.

Personally, I've become more convinced all the time that endeavoring to build healthy lives is made much better when founded on some basic principles of faith. I'm still not sure how important it is what exactly we believe, though I think conceding to some greater authority beyond ourselves has real merit, at least in placing ourselves in a more realistic universal context if nothing else.

I should mention that the trip to Dallas coincided with my son's birthday party, which totally sucked on many levels, not the least of which was getting Amy pissed at me. But I knew I had to go for two reasons. For one, Randall is a true friend and he would do the same for me in a second. Also, if I say I believe what I believe but then don't back it up with action when it really matters, then what the hell does it matter?

So I went to Dallas, joking along the way with Amy's dad that we were on a mission from God à la the Blues Brothers. But the deeper we got into it, the more we actually started to believe it. This is a bit of a divergence, but it's worth telling.

On the plane to Dallas, there was a particularly spunky African-American flight attendant who actually, at one point, smacked me in the back of the head. The funny thing was that I kind of liked it. She jawed back and forth with us the whole trip and finally offered us a couple of free drinks for being good sports. I passed, given that it was ten in the morning, and a shot that early not only sounds gross but it would knock me out for the rest of the day. Mark, on the other hand, explained that he didn't drink, which sparked a whole conversation about why we were on our way to Texas. By the time we touched down at Dallas/Fort Worth airport, she offered us her blessings and wished us Godspeed in our mission.

It kinda came out of the blue, smacking me in the head and then blessing me, but I'll take it wherever I can get it.

Then we got to the car rental place and another black woman behind the counter greeted us with, what would have been on any other day, a sort of creepy welcome. No one should be that happy to see a customer, especially when all they're doing is renting a car for a day, but she clapped her hands, got us some bottled water, and started asking about our trip. So we told her.

"Praise God!" she shouted. "I've been in ministry myself for five years. You're doing God's work here today." Far be it from me to argue, I guess. On our way out, she also offered a blessing and said she would be praying for us.

Again whether you believe in God or not, I don't think that having someone praying for you has ever done a bit of harm to anyone. So pray away.

The next morning while we were having breakfast at a diner down the street from Randall's sister's house, our waitress—also African-American—acted as if she had known us for years. And then, without mentioning a word about why we were there, she leaned over to Mark and, under her breath, said that he reminded her of her first sponsor.

In Twelve-Step speak, a sponsor is the person who has been through the program and now commits to helping new folks navigate sobriety. So of all the things she could have said, she mentions her Twelve-Step sponsor, less than an hour before we were headed into an intervention.

When we told her what we were going to do, I thought she might pass out right there in the middle of the restaurant. "My goodness, I got goose bumps," she said. "This is God's work happening today. You're on God's mission."

One black woman blessing your work is nice. Two is uncanny. Three is freakish and begins to seem beyond all coincidence.

So in my estimation, a life with God is no guarantee of picket fences; perfect, healthy families; and two-point-five kids with perfect teeth. The lives we inherit are messy, sometimes painful, and maddeningly inscrutable. The good news is our lives also are woven together. Thank God.

Our parents may screw us up six ways from Sunday or we may do more screwing up on our own, without parental assistance. But if we're open and if we at least believe that love is possible, whether you attach the face of God to the notion or not, it comes back in kind as you offer it up. Randall, broken as he is, offered himself freely and the bonds of love and friendship were the very connections that led us back to his side in his moment of greatest need.

And somewhere, in the middle of it all, grace showed her face, not once but three times.

CHAPTER 27

twitch

Daddy, we're going to kill Miles tomorrow. He's going to be dead. I wished him a merry Christmas, even though he'll have Christmas this year as an angel up in heaven.

—Mattias, 5 years

I've had this twitch in my left eye for over a month now. It started in my upper eyelid, tweaking my vision once every few minutes. Then one day, I woke up and it had migrated to the bottom eyelid. About a week later, it jumped back up to the top of my eye, though more aggressively, halfway closing my eye involuntarily, and often at the most inconvenient moments.

I had written it off as collateral damage related to our Thanksgiving plans. It started out with Amy's brother, Matt, deciding to come with his wife and two kids to Pueblo for the big day. By the time Thanksgiving actually arrived, we had upwards of thirty crowded in an L-shape of mix-and-match tables, from our dining room, around and through the living room to the front door.

I'm not what most would call overly hospitable. I'm all about having a couple of friends over for dinner, and even two families are generally manageable. But when you start getting into double digits, my anxiety level goes off the charts. Most of my stress manifested itself pre-Thanksgiving, and the day of there was nothing that a Xanax and a couple beers didn't help me get through. But the next day, and for several days afterward, the twitch remained.

"I think there's something else going on," said Amy, choosing her words carefully. I can always tell when an armchair diagnosis is to follow because she speaks as if every word is balanced on top of a tightrope.

"I know," I said, "I've got too much going on."

"No, that's not what I was thinking. You've been talking about writing your dad for a while, and you haven't done it. I think if you did—if you got off your chest whatever is following you around, that twitch might go away."

"Hmm," I knew she was probably right, but writing a letter to my dad, who had ignored any communication for several years, was not tops on my can't-wait-to-do list.

"There's something else," she said, looking a little sad. "I think you're hanging on to Miles because he's that last connection you have to that time in your life."

Ugh. It's always weird when someone else knows better what's going on in your head than you do. Miles is my nineteen-year-old cat who is clinging with one half-rotted tooth to the tail-end of his ninth life. He has lost much control over his orifices, he wails randomly at the wall, and he's stopped responding when I call to him. He was becoming so destructive in the house that we moved him and Lenny, the crappy other cat Amy brought into our marriage, to the basement where there's nothing but cement to defile.

We had consulted with a family member who is a vet, and she said Miles probably was suffering from hyperthyroidism and possibly some degree of kidney failure too. When asked about what to do with him, she basically gave me permission to let him go, and noted that living in the basement was no real quality of life anyway, for either animal.

I've known what I needed to do for a while, but Amy's right; I just haven't been ready to let him go. I got Miles from a department store window in the mall where I was working part-time at a bookstore during my senior year in high school. The local shelter put up a display at the store every Christmas to try to expedite adoptions, and I guess in my case it worked.

Come to think of it, it was almost exactly nineteen years to the day today when I brought him home. I guess there's some bizarre symmetry to putting him to sleep—or as Mattias likes to say, killing our cat—today, a week before Christmas.

I remember seeing the puffy little herd of cats in the display window during my lunch break and going straight back up to the store (this was way before cell phones) to call my mom and ask her about adopting one. My folks had just recently separated and I was living with my mom in a townhome, about ten miles from the house where we had lived previously with my dad. There were all sorts of emotional and logistical hurdles to clear that holiday season, given that it was the first time in my life that my folks would celebrate Christmas in separate places. It also was about eight months before I headed north to college, so needless to say, I felt a little bit rootless.

I guess my mom took some pity on my situation, and given that I had planned to move into my own apartment in college and would otherwise be alone, she greed to let me bring one home. I was never really a cat person, but I knew there was no way I could take a dog with me to college. A cat was self-sufficient enough that I could make it work, I figured, and lucky for me Miles was always more like a dog than a cat in his disposition.

At his peak, he weighed in at close to twenty pounds, lumbering lazily around to one sunny spot on the floor and then another until making his way back to the food bowl and the crapper. He'd snooze for hours on my lap as I studied and would always come when I called him. He even fetched on occasion, which is remarkable for a creature of the otherwise-aloof feline persuasion. He's been with me through at least eight moves, from Texas to Seattle and Colorado, through both conflicts in Iraq, through 9/11 and two major stock market crashes. He's been a part of my family almost twice as long as Amy, and by now he's lasted more than half of my life. So yeah, given his tenure, and especially the timing with which he arrived on the scene, I'd say he's been pretty important.

But now his fur is all matted and stained with God-knows-what. He stopped grooming himself a couple of years ago and once he moved into the basement, I'll admit that I gave up on trying to keep him cleaned up. He looks like he has cataracts and he stumbles whenever he walks, always looking a little bit like Gary Busey on a bender, weaving down Hollywood Boulevard.

So yeah, it's time. As of two o'clock this afternoon, he will cease to be a cat in the physical sense. We'll send him along his way.

I wasn't around when Amy told Mattias about the plan, but she told me later that he took it pretty hard. She held him for about fifteen minutes while he cried it out. I guess he's better at processing things emotionally and moving on, because by the time I got home from work, he walked straight up to me and announced that we were going to kill Miles, and that, following said killing, he would officially be dead.

Hey, we all work through grief in our own ways. He, like his mother, has a good cry and then talks the thing to death, while I exhibit physical symptoms and eventually get around to writing about it. Whatever works, I guess.

I figured I was on a bit of a roll, what with the cat-euthanizing spree under way, so I decided to go ahead and write the letter to my dad while I was inspired. First of all, I had resolved not to spend yet another Christmas dwelling on the absence of family, instead focusing on what I do have, and to do that I was pretty sure I needed to put my thoughts and feelings down on paper.

There's also the matter of my responsibility as a father and a husband. I've noticed, over the past few months, that this worry I carry around inside comes out in one way or another, and more often than not, the recipients of my little outbursts are those closest to me. I owe it to Amy and Mattias to unburden myself of this old family stuff, especially since they have so little to do with it anyway. I also owe it to baby Zoe, not to bring her into a world where the joy of her birth is clouded by my own inability to work through grief, conflict, and loss. It's not like whacking my cat and writing my dad an e-mail make me magically purified and able to parent without fault, but it helps remove some of those barriers that get built up over time between us and the rest of the world; this is particularly the case with men too.

So I wrote the letter and I sent it. Amy remarked about how quickly it all went down; I sat down after putting Mattias to bed and knocked it out in about fifteen minutes, then sent it off. She figured I'd let it simmer for a while or ask her to read over it before I e-mailed it, but pretty much, once I resolve to do something hard like that, it's a lot like ripping off a Band Aid; I don't really want to prolong it any more than necessary. Plus, I'd been thinking for a while about what to write, so it wasn't as if this was my first go-round with it.

I caught him up on a few of the highlights he's missed in the past few years. I let him know, just in case he hadn't heard from somewhere else by now, that he was going to be a grandpa again. I showed off a few of my achievements, since we all still want approval from our parents, no matter the circumstances. I told him that having to ask him to leave my in-laws' house a few years back was one of the most humiliating moments in my life and that if I had it to do over again, I would have left with him instead of staying behind and watching him leave alone. I told him I loved him and reiterated, as I did the night he left, that he's always welcome in our home.

That's it. Just over a page long, nothing eloquent or frilly. It won't go down as a great moment in literature, and frankly I don't even know if he'll read it. But I wrote it just to write it and not based on an expected outcome. I wrote it to hopefully get rid of this twitch in my eye. I wrote it to show my family, and I guess myself too, that part of being a man is dealing with your baggage head-on and not leaving a mess for others to deal with. I wrote it because he's my dad regardless of whether he's a part of our lives, and he deserves to know he's going to have a granddaughter. And I wrote it because, just like putting Miles to sleep, it's the right thing to do.

So why does doing the right thing suck so much sometimes? At least so far my eye has not twitched at all since I sent it. As far as Miles goes, I just have to trust that I'm doing what's right. That's the other challenge in being a grown-up: not having someone else to confirm for you which are the right choices and which are the wrong ones. If the twitchless eye is any indication though, I may be on the right track.

CHAPTER 28

in-laws

> Me: *Look, it's a full moon.*
>
> Mattias: *Oh yeah? What did they feed it?*
>
> —Mattias, 3 years, 4 months

It was a hell of a week. More specifically, Friday was a hell of a day. I was home from working up in Beulah, so we planned a whacking ceremony for my cat. For those who have never put an animal to sleep, it's surprisingly quick once they put the syringe in. Within a few seconds they have X's on their eyes. When Miles went, it was almost cartoonish, with his tongue lolling out and his eyes bugged open. I tried to close his eyes, like they do at the crime scenes on TV, but as soon as I did they'd pop right back open. So I settled for letting him stare at me with that vacant, I-give-you-nineteen-years-of-my-life-and-this-is-the-thanks-I-get glare.

Sucks being a pet.

About an hour before I took Miles to meet his maker, my dad e-mailed me back, which I was not ready for. He thanked me for my note, wished me luck with the new baby, and basically reiterated that he had no plans to be involved in our lives anymore. He even quoted scripture to me, about husbands and wives and cleaving or some stuff, and he quoted the Serenity Prayer, which is a kind of the cornerstone of Twelve-Step work:

> God, grant me the serenity
> to accept the things I cannot change,
> the courage to change the things I can,
> and the wisdom to know the difference.

He went with the first bit about accepting the things he could not change. But whereas in the Twelve-Step program, the unchangeable things they are talking about are external, with my dad he's talking about his own personality, as if it were carved out of granite. He recognizes that he has an abrasive tongue and comparable personality overall, but he takes sort of the Popeye philosophy: *I yam what I yam, and that's all that I yam.*

It's frustrating because I don't buy this as justification for walking away from your only son and only two grandchildren, but it's his choice and I really can't do much about that. Amy asked me if I thought I should take Mattias down to Dallas with me to see him, but I don't think it would do any good. When my dad's done, he's done. Period.

The one good thing about the timing of his letter was that it afforded me a two-for-one sob session at the vet's office. It was kind of nice to get them both out of the way as a package deal, especially since crying knocks me out for a couple days anyway and, as I've already mentioned, I got my quadrennial quota in for tears when I went to see Randall who, incidentally, is doing great in treatment and is headed home in a few days. So there's a little ray of sunshine warming the doo-doo pot a bit.

Guy logic tells you to deal with difficult stuff like this head-on, and in general I think that makes sense. The problem is that it leaves a residue or a series of emotional aftershocks that reverberate through the rest of your life, sometimes indefinitely, and definitely without any predictable pattern. It sucks for the people who actually do live with you because they get to bear the brunt of your mood swings, which actually have to do more with the dead cat and/or the absent parental unit. But since they're unavailable, your "family of choice" has to do.

I use the terms "family of origin" to refer to blood relatives and "family of choice" in reference to the people you marry, have kids with, make lifelong friends with, and so on. In some cases your family of origin also can be your family of choice, though not always. In my case, I am lucky to have a large, somewhat insane but very loving and vibrant family of choice. One of the best things about Mark Pumphrey, Amy's dad, is that he always has emotional room for one more. The bad thing is that he seems hell-bent on removing himself from the herd we call humanity.

At least the ways in which he chooses to nearly off himself—pretty much yearly—are great material for stories. Unfortunately for him, his son-in-law is a writer, so he has no cover. But these stunts of his are way too good to keep as quaint family anecdotes over holiday eggnog.

The first award-winning stunt took place a couple years ago, after Mark had an argument with his wife about something and he stormed out of the house toward his office at the church. On the way out the door, he grabbed a banana and chomped on it as he bounded down the front steps, convincing himself with every step of how right he was and how wrong his wife had been.

By the time he reached the street, he tossed the peel aside to help punctuate his conviction, looked up to check traffic, and promptly stepped directly on top of his own banana peel. Though I wasn't there, the way he recounts it is just like in the cartoons, where a character's feet fly completely out from under them, hovering inexplicably in midair for a moment before crash, all asses and elbows, to the ground.

What a way to go, Pumphrey, he said to himself as he pulled up to his hands and knees, only to look up toward an oncoming city bus. He made it to the curb before getting flattened by Denver's finest public transport, though it would not have surprised any onlookers if a piano or a safe had fallen from the sky at that moment, squishing him down into a pancake shape followed by him walking away like an accordion.

Possibly the best thing about this whole story is that he, being a minister, got many miles out of the metaphor of slipping on his own banana peel. Amy and I have milked it too, having used the story in a sermon and a newspaper column, respectively. Lately, the story well had been running a little dry, but thankfully the gods smiled on us all and made great material once again out of one of Mark's mishaps.

He and his wife, Mary Kay, are way into this timeshare system, having amassed a ton of points and so they take little trips out of town all the time. This last week, they took a couple of days up in the mountains, but on the way up their wiper fluid pump crapped out. Anyone who has traveled in the mountains in the winter knows that there's enough salt, sand, and other garbage on the highway that you can't make it more than a mile or two without decent wipers, so they made a quick stop and improvised.

Mary Kay grabbed one of the water bottles they had in the back and filled it with wiper fluid so she could reach outside and spray it on the windshield manually as needed. They made it to their destination just fine, and just before they headed back they decided to take in a scenic hike. And hiking, especially up at high altitude, can make anyone work up a serious thirst. Good thing they had plenty of water back at the car, right?

Mark hops in the driver's seat and, without so much as a glance behind him, grabs the first bottle he can reach and downs about half of the tasty beverage before taking pause to assess the curious nature of this water he's been ingesting.

"God," he grimaced, looking down at the bottle now only half-full of blue liquid, "what the hell did I just drink?"

"You didn't," Mary Kay said in disbelief. "Did you seriously just drink the wiper fluid?" Immediately, Mark leapt from the car and ran to the nearest snow bank, forcing himself to vomit as quickly and violently as he could. Cascades of blue sprayed east and west as he shoved his fingers down his throat. Mary Kay brought the original bottle around the front of the car, which was emblazoned with a large skull and crossbones, along with the grave warning that swallowing the stuff could cause blindness or even death.

"I think we should head to the hospital now," said Mark, postvomit.

One benefit to drinking poison is that you get hastily to the front of the line in the emergency room. The liability is that you get to explain, first to the emergency room staff and then to the chief hospital administrator, that you are neither suicidal nor married to a spouse with murderous tendencies. Then you have to explain, after eliminating the more scintillating possibilities, how it is that a grown man ends up downing several mouthfuls of windshield washer fluid.

They monitored him for a while to ensure that his vital signs remained stable and Mark, never missing an opportunity to tell on himself, called Amy to relay the events. "I've really done it this time," he said, recalling the morbid details.

Mark, like Miles, definitely has more than one life on his celestial line of credit. The man puts himself through some harsh, albeit creatively amusing, scenarios. Once again, he's lived to tell the tale, for which we are glad on many levels. Not only do we want to keep him around a good while longer, we also would really hate to have to shelve such a good story simply because his untimely demise got in the way.

People check out in lots of different ways. My dad's more of a fan of the clean break, while Mark's is more incremental and definitely more amusing. There are plenty of stories about parents worrying over their kids' self-destructive behavior and/or emotional distance, but what about when it's the other way around? There's only so much a kid can do about that. My focus is on not repeating the cycle. Seems to me I have a better chance of success with that than I do changing decades of ingrained behavior in my relatives.

CHAPTER 29

a-hole dad

> Mattias: *Dad, I forgive you.*
>
> Me: *But I didn't do anything wrong.*
>
> Mattias: *That's OK. I forgive you anyway.*
>
> —Mattias, 5 years, 1 month

Perhaps the biggest responsibility of a parent is to impart a worldview to your kids that reflects your values, so that once your kids are out making their own decisions, at least they have the benefit of your wisdom to call on if they choose to. It turns out, though, that sometimes we're our own worst parental enemies.

Take yesterday, for example, when I realized I'm a big, gigantic jerk of a dad.

I've still been recuperating from the emotional fallout of the past week's events and, as such, I haven't felt much like being around lots of people. So when Amy's family gathered for lunch in Pueblo, I passed. I did have lots of work to do, but the main impetus for me was that I was craving isolation, which is something entirely foreign to the Pumphrey clan.

My son, on the other hand, has never known a moment in his life when he didn't want to be at the center of activity. So Amy took him to the lunch and he proceeded to charm the crap out of everyone. I'm glad to see how socially adept he is, because one of my concerns in having kids to begin with was that they might inherit my antisocial gene. I think there's no concern about that with Mattias in the least.

They put him between Jed and Joe, two of his favorite people, so he was in uncle heaven. I guess at one point he leaned over to his uncle Joe and announced, unsolicited, that he adored him, to which Joe responded by giving him five bucks.

Now I love that Mattias is so unabashedly affectionate with people, but I do hope he doesn't equate kindness with compensation. That could get a little weird, walking up to strangers and relatives with a kind word on his tongue and hand eagerly extended. I don't see that kind of potential in him though, so I guess a little spoiling from his family can't hurt much.

As he tends to do, he was parading the cash around to anyone who would acknowledge it, including to me, as if it was the only five-spot ever minted. The problem is that about half the time, he loses the money before it makes it into his bank. So I offered to carry it for him while we were out running some errands later on. He asked for it back after a while and I explained that if he lost it, there were no refunds. I figured, though, that even losing the money was a lesson worth learning.

Sure enough, that evening at dinner, he dug into his pocket for his cash and found nothing. "Dad," he said, looking distressed, "I need my money back."

"I already gave it to you, buddy," I said, bracing for the inevitable fit to follow.

"No," he said, raising both the pitch and volume of his voice, "you have it."

"Remember how we talked about this?" I sat down with him, checking his pockets. "This is why I didn't want you to carry your own money. Once it's gone, it's gone, dude."

"I did NOT lose it!" he was pretty worked up at this point. "You had it, and YOU lost it!" His eyes got a little bit teary, though you could tell he was still trying to hold it together.

"Hey, don't blame me for losing your money," I said, trying to balance his distress with an even tone of voice. "Sometimes we lose stuff. It's no fun, but that's how we learn to be more careful."

"No," he stood up, shifting from plaintively desperate to confrontational, "YOU had it, YOU lost it, and I want it back!"

"All right," I rubbed my eyes, trying not to get hooked by his tirade, "that's enough. Go take a time out and think about how you're talking to daddy." He stomped over toward his Naughty Step, all the while grumbling audibly about my culpability and something about his displeasure for my stinkiness. I let it slide, as he was already being punished, but I let him know in no uncertain terms that if he escalated his name-calling, he'd be spending some time in the gulag, also known as the car bed in his room.

After a few minutes, he got the frustration out of his system and I let him out of the penalty box. As I try to do after his punishment, I gave him a hug and tried to talk him through why he got in trouble and how he might avoid it the next time. He played along, if for no other reason than to get me to shut up so he could go back to watching the animated Christmas special that was on TV.

The best thing I've observed about folks like my wife and Mattias, who seem to wear their emotions out there for all to see, is that they get over stuff pretty quickly. After a couple of commercial breaks, Mattias hopped off the couch and came over to my chair. "Dad," he said, giving me a squeeze, "I love you, and I forgive you."

"Thanks buddy," I said, hugging him back, "but do you know what it means to forgive someone?"

"Kind of," he said, staring at me with his big, blue saucer eyes. It's a damn good thing this kid is so stinking cute; it may well add to his lifespan.

"It means you're not staying upset at someone for something they did wrong."

"OK," he said, giving me another hug, "then I forgive you."

"But I didn't do anything wrong," I said, careful not to bring up the money specifically, for fear of starting another emotional conflagration I'd just as soon avoid.

"I forgive you anyway," he smiled, and went back to his TV show.

Fair enough. Who am I, after all, to dissuade him from offering peace in his own way, even if it's a little bit misdirected?

A couple hours later, as I was getting ready for bed, I emptied my pockets onto the bathroom counter and tucked up in the corner of my right-hand pocket was a crumpled up five-dollar bill. I stared at the object in utter shame.

"What's the matter," Amy asked. I held up the bill. "You're kidding," was all she said.

"I'm such a knob," I said, setting his money down.

"So what are you going to do?"

"I'm going to apologize to him of course."

"Poor guy," she frowned. "Five-year-olds just have no leverage to argue."

"All right," I said. "Thanks, but I already feel like enough of an asshole."

"You should ask him what you can do to make it right."

"Yeah," I said, "good idea to basically open the door to a kid to let him exploit the moment."

"Well, that's what we teach him to say."

"No," I corrected her, "that's what you teach him to say. I think an apology and admitting you're wrong is good enough. I hate apologizing as it is."

"Really? I didn't know that about you."

"In the Piatt clan," I said, "the typical M.O. was just to ignore the transgression for a while until you could just pretend like it never happened."

"Nice," she shook her head.

"Hey, I didn't say I was going to do it, but I'm sure as hell not going to go wake him up to apologize." He was still asleep when I left for work the next morning, so I got to carry it around a little longer, which is awesome for a guy already feeling off-center about my own parental issues. I guess it's a healthy lesson in humility for me and, at the same time, it was a real eye-opener in retrospect to realize he was forgiving me even though he knew I had his money the whole time, and for all he knew, I had lost it, leaving him with no recourse.

Talk about mixed emotions. I'm both proud to be his dad and feeling like a total schmuck for putting him through all of that. Amy's right; this one probably is going to cost me a little.

Being the little five-year-old saint that he is, I could hardly finish apologizing before he was hugging and forgiving me. "It's OK dad, I forgive you, *again*. I forgive you every time, and plus, even though it's not Valentine's Day, you can be my Valentine every day."

"That's very sweet," I said, both grateful for his mercy and even more embarrassed about my faux pas. "Thanks buddy."

"But dad," he said, pulling back and looking me in the eye, "I will remember this and you will too. Every Christmas eve until you die, you will remember this five dollar bill."

Part of good parenting, from what I can tell anyway, is modeling how to deal well with flaws. Along the way in my childhood, I got the mistaken impression that being a good parent meant presenting an aura of flawlessness, which of course can't be sustained forever. I remember the grave disappointment I experienced when I realized my parents not only weren't right all the time, but that they were actually just as messed up as everybody else. It's a harsh realization, much like learning the truth about Santa and other mythologies upon which we hang our youthful hopes, and although I'm not set on a mission to overwhelm my kids with premature disillusionment, I also don't want them to expect a world that can't deliver. Part of my job, then, is to admit when I'm a screw-up.

The best news is that at his age and given his naturally loving disposition, he's already inclined to forgiveness, even when I'm not ready to accept it. I can only hope to learn from such grace, compassion, and I guess you could call it wisdom. At least for today, the teacher has become the student. Despite appearances, Mattias is actually the better person in many ways and I have a hell of a lot to learn. I could take this as a major blow to my own ego, but I prefer to see it as a gift to get to learn from someone so relatively new to the human race.

Take wisdom wherever you can get it, I say. That includes kids who forgive you, even before you know you need it.

CHAPTER 30

pointers

Here mom, I'll say something funny and you write it down in here.

—Mattias, 4 years, 9 months

I've made a conscious effort not to make this book a how-to advice book for expectant parents. First of all, what the hell do I know? Second, there are already plenty of books out there about how to handle pregnancy by people way more knowledgeable than I am. I'm just some guy who decided to work out my neuroses on the page and you happen to be reading it. That hardly makes me an expert on anything.

That said, I feel like I have to at least lay out a few things for people—especially guys—who will never be caught dead picking up another parenting book, so this may be as close to parental self-help as you'll ever get. So here are a few things to know, consider, or avoid during the pregnancy process:

Worry—You may think that once you get pregnant, you can stop worrying. But pretty much, once you've joined your little swimmer to that egg, your worry-free days are done. As a friend of ours put it, you worry about getting pregnant until you are, then you worry about staying pregnant. Once the baby's viable, you worry about the birth. After the birth, you worry about every grunt and spurt the baby issues. Once they walk, you worry about them falling down, and so on. This continues until either they or you die, whichever comes first.

Remodeling—Guys, you will pay for remodeling in your house, even if you move into a house with a nursery already intact that was designed by Martha Stewart herself. Chicks have to feel like they're making their own unique mark in order to be responsible parents, so be ready. Oh, and in case it's not already self-evident, your opinions about furniture, color, and everything else amount to zero. Just buy and carry stuff as requested.

Cravings—Yes, your wife will have cravings and no, you cannot predict what, how much, or when. Always have a ten spot next to your keys for when—not if—you are asked to make a late-night run. Consider eliminating anything resembling the following phrases at least for the next nine months, if not forever:

"Are you sure you should eat that?"

"Maybe the doctor should check again to make sure we're not having twins."

"Hey let's see who weighs more."

"Hey honey, could you grab me a beer?"

"But you never ate that before."

Your Role—Get to know your responsibility for the coming months now to avoid any retribution that might render your reproductive organs useless in the future, or for which you may find yourself sleeping in the dog's kennel. In general, there is nothing you will do in the coming year that is as important as what your wife is doing, so drop excuses like, "I was busy" or "I'm just swamped" from your lexicon. As a female friend of mine put it to her husband after he commented on how much she napped: "I grew a human being inside my body today. What the hell did you do?"

Staring—People are going to stare at your wife, be they male or female. If you're the possessive type, get over it. Yes, it's reasonable to run interference when strangers come up and try to touch your wife's belly, and trust me they will. But they'll stare as if they've never seen a distended uterus before. Some people will even comment, rather loudly, about your wife's shape, as if she were encased behind some mobile, invisible soundproof glass. Avoid the urge to hit them in the face, unless they say something like the graphic designer buddy of mine who informed Amy he kind of had a fetish for preggos. Then swing away.

Labor—Though it might seem like a straightforward concept, there are lots of different kinds of labor. There are Braxton-Hicks contractions, which happen throughout the pregnancy. These do not mean anything is wrong; on the contrary, it's the woman's body's way of getting ready for the Big Game. There's also false labor, which generally happens closer to the birth, increasing in frequency the further along she is. Just one healthy contraction should not send you bolting for the emergency room. Usually you want to wait until she's having them regularly, at least every five minutes for about an hour. Her belly will be hard as granite and she'll usually feel the pain radiating from her lower back toward the front.

If you're not sure, call your doctor, but don't be that annoying guy who calls about every little thing. Remember that you want the physicians on your side once you actually need them, because after you're admitted to the hospital for the real deal, you're more or less a piece of cattle for them to move through the system. Make friends and influence people, which begins with being a big boy and realizing that childbirth is hard; that's why they call it "labor."

Birthing Options—I'm no doctor, but our first experience with Amy's labor being induced totally sucked. Clearly Mattias was not ready to be born yet, which is not exactly shocking since it was three days before his due date, but they scheduled her labor out of convenience for the doctor and the hospital. By then Amy was more than ready to get the beast out of her body and we didn't know any better, so we agreed. Unfortunately, he had not moved into the proper position and her contractions came so hard and fast after the Pitocin was administered that he got forced unnaturally into the birth canal. This time, there's no way anyone's shooting Amy full of that junk unless her life or Zoe's depends on it.

Same goes with planned C-sections. Some physicians and hospitals push this option because they have more control, but always remember: it's your baby and, in your wife's case, it's her body. Don't let someone carve on her just because it works better for them. Don't be afraid to strong arm the docs a little bit if they get pushy too. Women's bodies have known what to do without a doctor's help for millions of years, so don't let them fool you into believing they know your wife's body better than she does. Granted, such procedures have saved plenty of lives, but sometimes a doctor's faith in medicine reaches religious levels.

That having been said, make sure you follow your wife's lead on birthing options. Be man enough to express your opinions, but also be smart enough to know when to shut up. You may think natural childbirth is a great idea, but it's not you squeezing the kid out in the end so, as is the best bet in most cases involving pregnancy, defer to her.

Sex—If you thought you didn't have the upper hand in your sexual relationship before, you just lost what few chips you had. Pregnancy makes some women hornier than ever, while others would just as soon rip your weiner off as let you near her with it. Oh, and sometimes those are both the same woman. It's a tricky balance though, because if you avoid all intimacy entirely, this will likely feed into her perception that she's not sexy while pregnant, and hence the penis-removing commences anew.

Your best bet is to compliment her sincerely and often, but not too often, offer physical contact in the form of foot and back rubs, and then wait for the "go" signal. If it never comes, well, you remember what that's like, right?

Registering—I guarantee that the first time you register for a baby, you'll sign up for tons of stuff you don't need and you'll forget lots of other things you'll wish you had. Talk to a friend who's already had a kid and ask them what the can't-live-without items are, such as Boppys, Super Swaddlers, Bumbo Seats, and all the other crap no other generation had but now we suddenly can't live without. And if their kid has outgrown it, don't feel weird about borrowing their gear. Most of it hardly even gets broken in before your baby is too big for it, so take it willingly and then pass it along.

Though I'm not a big fan of opposite-sex shopping sprees, I do recommend you join your wife when registering. Places like Target that offer the little radar gun are great, allowing you just to click on the stuff you want instead of writing it all down by hand. You can also update your list online, which you'll need to do since some people will buy you stuff from other stores or they'll keep getting you stuff after your registry says you have more than enough. Also, keep your gift receipts and take back what you're not going to use. Better to trade in that pink and yellow plaid jumper for a box of diapers than to worry too long about hurting someone's feelings. Get what you need.

Showers—There's this phenomenon recently of throwing couples' showers. Some of these are great, but most of them suck and you'll wish you never went, unless you're into obnoxious party games and watching your wife open presents for two hours that everyone will exclaim are either "precious" or "adorable."

There is one simple screening that always will help you determine if this is the real kind of shower you want to be a part of: will there be beer served? If so, make sure it's scheduled on a day with a sporting event on TV, invite your friends into the other room for a cold one, and consider yourself a part of the festivities. Otherwise, stay very, very far away.

Dates—Remember that even if you're not getting any, you still need time together as adults. One of the biggest pitfalls new parents make is forgetting that they are a couple first and parents second. This doesn't mean you love your kids any less; it just means you recognize that your marriage has to be a priority or else your parenting will be severely compromised by a mediocre relationship, regardless of how great of a dad you are.

Set the precedent before the kid comes to keep at least one night a week as sacred couple time. If you have a parent or friend, plan ahead for babysitting. If not, hire a college student or trade off nights with other friends who have kids. It's harder to plan time alone once you have kids and if you're not already in the habit, you'll realize later that it's been months since you've been on a date. Meanwhile you sit around wondering why you and your wife only talk about your kids.

It's not complicated. You didn't get married without dating first, so why would you expect that maintaining a healthy relationship is any different?

Advice—Here's the ironic part of the chapter; my advice to you is generally to ignore the advice of others. Most of it is based in nothing but one person's own anecdotal experience, and most of it contradicts someone else's advice. That's not to say that you can't learn from other peoples' experience and especially from their mistakes, but opinions about pregnancy, childbirth and raising kids are like assholes: everybody's got one and no one wants to have anything to do with anyone else's.

Perhaps most important to remember, especially if you have an attention span like me and are lucky to hold on to two points at most from any given thing you read, remember this:

1. Your child is unique, special, and amazing.
2. So is everyone else's kid.

Though it's hard at times to reconcile these two truths, keeping them both in some sort of healthy balance is fundamental to becoming at least a less-than-crappy parent.

Good luck.

CHAPTER 31

wait, there's more

She is just so beautiful. I think I'll keep her forever.

—Mattias, 5 years, 2 months

It was just before four in the morning on Friday when Amy came up the stairs to the attic where I was sleeping.

"I think it's time," she said between breaths.

"Time for what?" I was still bleary from sleep and was clearly missing the obvious.

"The time," she said, "time to go to the hospital."

"Oh shit, that time," I rolled out of bed and to my feet, grasping for my glasses. "How far apart are they?"

"Three minutes, mostly," she said, "sometimes four. Here's another one." She grimaced and leaned forward against the railing.

"How long have you had them?" I asked. Women can have pretty strong contractions for twenty or thirty minutes without actually going into full-on labor. But usually, if they get up and move around or just wait it out, they'll go away in less than an hour.

"They started at 3:15," she said, "so almost an hour. I figure I'd just know and it feels like this is it, but the last thing I want is to be one of those women who runs to the hospital at the first sign of pain only to be sent home again."

"Well," I said, pulling a hat over my bed head, "what do you want me to do?"

"I don't know," she said. We stared at each other for a few seconds, as if some divine signal would drop from the sky and guide us through our ignorance. No such luck.

"Let's go get the rest of our stuff ready, and we'll see if they keep going." Amy must have been a boy scout in the past life, because when it comes to packing, she's more prepared than a Mormon for the apocalypse. All her hospital bag lacked was a few toiletries and the MP3 player. I, on the other hand, had not stopped to consider that I would be going to the hospital too, and that I might need some things as well. Amy decided to try to calm the contractions with a warm shower, so I took the opportunity to throw a few things in a bag.

"Just knock on the glass every time you have another one," I said. I had started writing down the time of each contraction along with a pain rating, on a scale one of to ten, to see if they were getting stronger or closer together. About every two to three minutes, another one hit.

"I don't know," she said through the shower door, "should we call the doctor?"

"Well, they're pretty close together," I said, "but what the hell do I know?"

"What if it ends up being a false alarm?"

"Tell you what," I picked up the phone, "I'll call. That way, if it's not the real deal, you can blame your worrywart husband." She didn't try to stop me, so I made the call. I got the midwife's pager, so I punched in my number and waited. Four or five contractions later, she had not responded, and I was getting a little bit pissed. "Let me call someone to come watch Mattias," I grabbed my phone again. "I say we go ahead to the hospital."

Mattias was sleeping in his room with his cousin, Miko, and we were not exactly excited about the prospect of dragging two little guys out of bed, through the emergency room, and up to the maternity ward, only to possibly witness the most gruesome event of their lives. Unfortunately, Miko's dad's phone was broken and his mom's was turned off, as was his sister's.

"We're having a baby and everyone's on sabbatical." We finally got hold of our friend, Audrey, who came from across town to run point at the house. Since we were less than two blocks from the hospital, and given that the parking garage was almost a block from the emergency room, we decided it made sense to walk.

"I wonder if anyone can guess what we're going to do," I said, holding Amy's arm as she had another contraction. Here we were, this goofy couple, one of whom is clearly bursting with child, walking down the street just before five in the morning with bags trailing behind us. We must have been quite a sight. "I'll bet you make it just to that curb before you have another contraction," I said. They were coming like clockwork and I was paying close enough attention that I could actually predict them within about five seconds. It was a fun little game, to try to guess when the next one would come, and it helped keep our minds off the possibility of any of a million things that could go wrong.

We showed the emergency room attendant all of Amy's preadmittance paperwork and they ushered her straight up to Labor and Delivery in a wheelchair.

"I'd really rather walk," she said. "It hurts more to sit down."

"Sorry," said the orderly, "hospital policy." There are many ironies about how hospital care is antithetical to patient needs or wishes, and this was one of those times. "Had a lady last week," she continued, "who gave birth right inside the CAT scan machine. Kinda cracked down on the whole wheelchair thing after that."

By the time the nurse on the maternity ward checked Amy, her cervix was already dilated six centimeters and she was fully effaced. In lay terms, this meant she was definitely, without question, for real, honest-to-God in labor. At first, I was relieved that we hadn't cried wolf, but then it hit me: oh mother, we're having a baby today.

It had taken until about six in the morning to get admitted and up to the room, and unless you're spraying blood from some body part, hospital time is about half the speed of normal life, at best. The contractions kept coming, and still no doctor and no midwife. They let us know Amy's doctor had been called, and about forty-five minutes to an hour later, they told us she had called to say she was just jumping into the shower and would be in soon.

"What the hell?" I fretted, watching the lines on the monitors spike up in jagged peaks as her contractions increased in intensity. "No one around here is in a hurry." Of course, they are used to delivering upwards of a dozen babies every day, so another woman in labor is no big thing, but to us it's one of only two we ever plan to experience, and we'd be damned if things were going to work out the way they did the first time.

An epidural is the type of medication a woman usually has to help with labor pain, but if it's given too early, it can seriously delay labor. Given too late, it doesn't take effect in time, so there's a window during which you have to decide whether or not to have one. Amy's doctor still had not arrived when Amy reached the point of trying to decide, which sucked because we really wanted her to help us make up our minds—as if she could know. By the time Amy was at eight centimeters—the final stage being ten—she was pretty damn sure she wanted the epidural, but she was close to the point of no return by then.

"It might slow your labor," said a nurse, "and it might stretch things out." There's also the matter of increasing the odds of having to have a cesarean-section delivery with an epidural, so amid these agonizing pains she's having to revisit her birth plan and make critical decisions while a human being the size of a couple of cantaloupes tried to make its way out of her.

I have to say, I admire her commitment to having a baby vaginally because she declined the epidural, opting instead to take the pain full-on. They did add a little bit of anesthetic to her IV drip and they squirted something akin to Novocain into her girl parts, but otherwise it was her, the baby, and a load of pushing between her and the end of the road.

"I want this f***ing thing out!" she hollered between contractions. "I want my mom too." By this time, the doctor had arrived, scrubbed up, and in a matter of less than a minute, had assembled every birthing tool on the wing, along with a cadre of nurses all staring at my wife's genitals. Turns out that the slow pace of hospital life is just a cover; they actually do know what is going on once it comes down to actual game time.

While the doctor was down between her thighs, Amy let out another howl. "No more noise!" shot the doctor. "I don't want to hear any more. Just breathing. Every time you yell, you take energy away from pushing. So when I tell you to, pull these legs back toward your head, breathe, and push as hard as you can until I tell you to stop. But NO MORE NOISE!" This doctor was half nazi and half ninja. What a badass.

It was right about this time that Amy's water broke. They call it "water" because words really can't describe the semigelatinous, mucousy, bloody concoction that oozed out in relatively large quantities. It was gross, but if it doesn't break, the baby can't be born, so I swallowed the puke creeping up the back of my throat and got back to my job.

Amy listened to her doc and did as instructed. As she began to feel the urge to push, which the female body amazingly knows to do just at the right time, I grabbed one leg by the heel. I can't remember exactly who had her other leg at this point because everything started to blur together, but by then her mom had made it from New Mexico, having driven at near lightspeed from the moment we called her earlier in the morning. Also in attendance were Amy's aunt, Rita—the one who introduced us in the first place—and her stepmom, Mary Kay, who is a nurse. My mom was still two days away so she'd miss the big party, but given the chaos, mingled with blood and far too many other fluids, I'd say she didn't miss the good parts.

At 9:13, with one final bloody push, baby Zoe Marie Piatt squirted out into the doctor's arms, followed by some more things that definitely would not be defined as "baby."

Resting her on my wife's chest, they handed me a pair of scissors to cut the umbilical cord, which is a strange metaphor in my opinion. Though it's meant to include the father in the birthing experience, there's something strangely dark about being the one severing the connection between mother and child. It's a necessary step, and one of many to come, but it's sort of hard to be the first one to sever the line. That and a healthy spray of cord blood squirted up my arm when I cut it, which was way nasty.

They handed her to me, thankfully discarding all the nonbaby stuff. And in that moment, something happened to me that would prevent me from ever being the same again for the rest of my life. As I watched her gasp for her very first lungful of air, I felt my own heart pouring into her. It was as if, in that moment, my hands had only been created to hold her, my eyes could see nothing other than her face, and my heart already had a perfectly formed space, shaped specifically for her, into which she perfectly and immediately fit.

Right at that moment would have been the time to ask me for the car keys, had she had the forethought to do it. I'd have given her anything in the world. How could I love someone so much that I'd just met a few moments before? Sure, the cynical side of me knows there's a chemical reaction that takes place to help ensure the parents will bond with the child and, therefore, will care for them. But there's more going on than good chemistry. For those willing to acknowledge it, God is right there, in that violent, chaotic moment of creation.

It's almost like a voice from somewhere whispered, "Let there be," and the next thing you know, there's baby Zoe in my arms. What a miracle; there's no other word to describe it.

* * *

Mattias is a big fan of infomercials these days. He dragged me into the living room from the kitchen the other day to watch a commercial for something called Mighty Putty, which is basically the same epoxy you can buy in any hardware store except that they make it look like the sexiest, most exciting and amazing product in the universe on TV. My son goes for the pitch every time.

"Look dad," he said, "you can fix a mug with it, or a leaky pipe, or even a broken chair!"

"But we don't have any of that broken stuff," I said.

"Yeah, but it can pull a truck," he protested.

"We don't have a truck either, dude."

"But wait," he grabbed my arm with one hand, pointing at the screen with the other, "there's more!" Ah yes, the telltale closing argument of every infomercial: "Wait, there's more!"

One of my worries about having another kid was making room. There was the physical issue of rooms and beds and such, but we got past that. Then there's the matter of time, money, and other logistics of child raising. But in all honesty, there are plenty of people in the world who raise way more children on way less money than we make, so that's a hard argument against kids.

The real issue comes down to emotional reserves. After opening yourself completely to a wife and a son, just how much further can the human heart stretch, especially one that's got its share of footprints still relatively fresh on it? Then all of a sudden . . .

Wait, there's more!

You just have enough. Love, it so happens, is an infinitely renewable resource. In fact it's the only commodity I know that multiplies when shared. My love for Zoe, though I'm still learning exactly what it is, is no less real or intense than the love I have for Amy or Mattias, but it's also distinctly different. She's never uttered a word, and our lives together include only a few bleary moments, yet my love for her is perfect.

CHAPTER 32

long overtime

I have a rash on my butt. I'm pretty sure it's cancer.

—Mattias, 5 years, 2 months

"Nothing goes in your vagina for six weeks," the doctor looked up from stitching Amy back together right after the birth. "Nothing."

I hate her so much.

If you think kids are a romantic buzzkill, you could not be more right, at least for the month and a half following childbirth. Your wife's boobs get gigantic, but touching them risks losing a digit, and aside from the pain you might inflict with sex, trying anything while things are still returning back to their normal state is kind of like throwing a nickel down a mine shaft anyway.

Aside from these "minor" setbacks, the family is great. I got the week following Zoe's birth off work for family medical leave, and Amy has three months of maternity time, though some in the church are pretty much convinced the building will crumble to the ground in that time. We've had tons of friends and family filing in and out of the house to ogle the new arrival, and to shower some needed attention on big brother too. As I sit here on the couch, basking in the luxury of personal reflection, I realize this is the first moment of real, wakeful silence I've had in about seven days. And for an introvert like me, the lack of solitude is a little bit like depriving me of oxygen after a while.

Mattias, on the other hand, feeds on crowds like rocket fuel. He's more animated than Roger Rabbit on speed, part of which is just his personality, but it also has to do with his way of dealing with change: I retreat and hide, while he puts on a Broadway show. If he didn't have my eyes, I might wonder if he was my kid sometimes.

One of his favorite things lately—big surprise—is to be held like a baby and act a lot like Zoe. Works for her, right? So we'll indulge him to some degree, though I prefer to give him props for doing more age-appropriate things like giving himself a bath and clearing his dishes. In reality though, he's still a little guy at heart, and even though he's reading full sentences, can tell the harmonic frequencies of train whistles, and has an encyclopedic knowledge of alternative music, he's still figuring out what it means to be something other than a baby in the world.

The long-term dependence we have on our parents is pretty much unique to human beings. While other offspring are shoved out of the nest after a few days and others literally hit the ground running, lest they get eaten, our progeny hang around for about eighteen years at least, and some forget they're ever supposed to leave. It's part of the trade-off of being the most emotionally and cognitively complex organisms in the known universe, I guess.

The butt-cancer comment at the top of the chapter came when we were getting him ready for bed the other night. The two things that seem to irk Mattias more than anything are that he has to go to school while Zoe stays here and that he has to go to bed while she stays downstairs. We've tried to explain that we have to watch her all the time right now and that he has other benefits of his age that she lacks, but in the moment, he feels like he's getting screwed. So I guess he decided he needed to invent a case of anal tumors to get our attention.

It reminds me of Ralphie from the movie *A Christmas Story*, who dreams of punishing his parents with crippling guilt someday for washing his mouth out with soap by appearing on their doorstep, completely blind.

"What brought you to this lowly state?" wailed Ralphie's dad. "Was it something we did?"

"It was . . . soap poisoning," he proclaims dramatically, as they prostrate themselves at his feet, eliciting a wily grin from Ralphie. And sure, who hasn't thought of punishing their folks at one time or another with some illness for which they are responsible? Talk about sweet revenge. And while Mattias may have to undergo a few sacrifices and adjustments to make room for Zoe in our lives, I'm not claiming culpability for his imaginary ass-cancer.

Overall, this pregnancy, delivery, and postnatal time has been easier in pretty much every way. I almost hesitate to write this down because the chances that Mattias will read this some day are good, and being a C-section baby with my own share of issues, I know I carried some guilt around for many years about putting my parents through a lot. But it's not like the babies have a choice. It's kind of like those parents who lay the pathos on their kids, talking about how much they sacrificed for them. Well, guess what? You didn't consult them before birthing them, so shut up.

Anyway, Zoe has been super easy so far, relatively speaking at least. She only cries when she's hungry or has to fart, and at six days old, she's already sleeping five or six hours at a time at night. He heart murmur, which they identified right after her birth, has disappeared on its own, as has her jaundice. The fact that Amy's recovery from a natural birth is much easier means she can help a lot more with both Mattias and the baby, which is a load off for me.

Part of why this go-round has been easier, though, is also because we know a little bit more about what we're doing. We're hardly perfect, but with the second kid, I'm already aware of worrying a lot less about screwing little things up. I don't jump out of my chair every time she squaws or gurgles, and I have a theory that part of why she sleeps so well is that the overall vibe in the house is more chilled out than when Mattias was born. So it's a bit of a chicken-or-the-egg argument, but either way we're more intentional about enjoying every moment we can with this new family we've made, rather than worrying quite so obsessively about screwing it up.

I started this book nine months ago with a title that would imply I had a lesson to learn in this experience. From the outset, it would seem that the lesson for me, being the one who wasn't so sure about having another kid, was how to keep myself out of this sort of mess in the future. But through this process, I've learned a lot of other things, not the least of which is that I think I can handle a four-person family without going bat-shit crazy. Some of the other things I've picked up are as follows:

- I've learned that fear is a barrier to a full life but that love is stronger.
- I've learned that I have a greater capacity for parenting, among other things, than I realized.
- I've realized that even though this world is full of disappointments, a new baby breaks through it all with the purest kind of joy, without doing much of anything except existing.
- I learned that I have to wait six weeks for sex or her doctor will kill me and that it's one of nature's cruel jokes to make her boobies so big and yet I can't touch them.

- I've learned that although I think I can handle being a new dad at age thirty-seven after all, I sure as hell don't want to make this a habit into my forties.
- I've learned that doing something that terrifies you isn't such a bad thing.
- I've learned how to at least pretend to be an adult, even when I still feel like a child inside sometimes.
- I've learned that the things I'm missing in order to be a part of this family, like late-night gigs and more time to write, are worth missing.
- I've learned that people crave an excuse to celebrate life, and that sharing your baby with them is a gift to them, even if it's a little bit inconvenient for you.
- I've learned never to trust a baby fart.
- I've learned the difference between a cry that says "I'm hungry," or "I'm tired," and one that says "hold me, just because."
- Finally, I have learned that you cannot die either from lack of sleep or from excessive exposure to vomit.

None of these presents any particularly novel revelation to the world, but some of this sort of wisdom, though available to all of us, is only realized through parenting, I believe. There's nothing wrong with deciding not to have kids, mind you, but although most childless couples cite other things they hesitate to sacrifice, they can't entirely know what they're giving up without a child of their own.

So one of my little swimmers pulled a Greg Louganis and triple-flipped his way into a willing egg, and that moment of weakness transformed itself into a beautiful baby girl. I can't say if I had it to do all over again I wouldn't be just as neurotic about the prospect of more kids, but I've decided she's a keeper. Mattias may not be so sure yet, but I'm pretty confident he has such a big heart that he'll find plenty of room for her in it. Amy's blissed-out in baby-land and I'm still finding time between the feedings, the diaper changes, and trips to the store for wipes to keep writing.

I'm not sure what anyone else would call it, but I call it a full life. I couldn't ask for anything else.

a.k.a. tying up loose ends,
a.k.a. killing the goalie

I'm thrilled to have Zoe in our lives. All of my concerns about worry overwhelming love and minutiae superseding the bigger picture of family thankfully were unwarranted. I should have known the love would come. I'm so crazy about this little girl it's stupid.

That said, there's no way in hell I want another one.

Though I'm glad Amy was able to deliver naturally and that there were few to no complications, it leaves me with no way to avoid going under the knife myself.

Amy is done with the pill; that much is abundantly clear. And unless I want the current sex drought to linger into my retirement years, it's incumbent upon me to do something about it. First, I checked with insurance to see what part of a vasectomy would be covered. Even though we have major medical policies with huge deductibles, I hoped that it would at least knock out a big chuck of the annual portion that fell to us, getting us closer to actually getting some benefits, but they don't cover a penny. Guess they don't really care how many kids we have since they also don't offer maternity coverage. Every new addition to the family unit is just another insured on the policy, so why encourage responsible family planning?

The first place I called wasn't even sure what they charged, which I thought was a little weird. It was almost like they wanted a peek in my wallet before they quoted me a price, pushing to set up a consult, for which they would naturally charge me. Scratch that one off the list.

I went through several others without luck, but finally got a referral from a friend. He sent me to Dr. F. who is close to seventy years old, and by his own count, has done more than two thousand of these procedures in his career. As I'm not a fan of offering up my genitals for trial runs, this sounded pretty good to me. Plus he charged nine hundred bucks, which—although it still seems outrageous for one short office visit and a thirty-minute in-office procedure–was the best deal I'd found.

Generally, a vasectomy isn't the kind of thing you want to bargain-shop for, but given this guy's experience and considering we're paying out-of-pocket for the whole thing, price does play a role. And at $900 for a half-hour gig, it's not like these are Walmart prices anyway.

The older Mattias gets, the more he overhears and absorbs. We can't spell anything anymore without him decoding it. I speak occasionally in broken Spanish to Amy, but he's learning that too. Most times I just give up and accept that he's a part of the conversation.

"Why are you going to the doctor, dad?" he asked, playing the Wii while eavesdropping on our chat about my research.

"I have to have a doctor check out my guy parts."

"Why?" he kept flicking away at the buttons on his remote.

"Because mom and dad are done making babies."

"How come?"

"Do you want more brothers or sisters?" I asked.

"I dunno."

"Well," I said, "we're pretty sure we don't so I'm going to take care of it."

"How do you do that?" he stopped and turned toward me. Clearly he wasn't going to be satisfied with generalities. He knew, more or less, how babies were made, but this whole how-to-stop-making-babies was new information.

"The doctor helps the sperm stay inside my body so they can't fertilize any of mommy's eggs," I said, continuing to take baby steps toward the truth while trying to spare him the gruesome details.

"You can stop them?" he asked. "How?"

Fine, I thought, *he wants to know, I'll tell him.*

"The doctor goes in with a knife and cuts my testicle sack open, pulls out the little tubes that connect the testicles to my penis, cuts them in half, and burns the ends with a little iron so the sperm are stuck in there for good." The boy's eyes looked like they might keep growing until they completely engulfed his entire head.

"You might bleed," he whispered in awe.

"Yeah, a little bit," I said.

"Maybe you'll die," he said, worry gnarling up his young face.

"I know it sounds really gross," I said, "but it's not that big of a deal. They do it all right there in the doc's office, and I can even drive myself home after."

"I don't want anyone cutting on my testicles," he said, stepping back away from me as if I was the one with the scalpel.

"Join the club, dude."

I remember the first time I drove a car. I was so excited and paranoid at the same time that I could hardly think. Over time though, it's become pretty much second nature. It's not until I have a kid in the car to ask a thousand questions about how it's done that I realize there's actually quite a lot to it.

I like to think that Dr. F.'s cavalier approach to vasectomies is kind of like the way I approach driving. The guy's sliced four thousand vas deferens in his career—though there was one dude with three vas deferens—so let's say four thousand and one. But for me, they're the only two I've got, so I'm a little bit concerned about how it all goes down. I suppose the conversation we had during the consult was supposed to reduce my anxiety, but it actually had the opposite effect.

"You hear all kinds of stories from other guys," said the doctor, rolling back and forth on his backless chair. "I don't really know why guys like to pass along these overdone horror stories, but they do."

Really? What horror stories? I thought. But I just nodded as if I knew what he meant.

"Despite what you hear, you do not experience impotence or a reduction in sex drive afterwards."

Whew, that's a relief.

"You won't experience phantom pain in your scrotum for years following the procedure."

Hell, I'd hope not.

"And your testicles will not swell up like melons."

Now what is this guy talking about? How do stories like that even get started? Maybe some guy, somewhere *does* have balls the size of cantaloupes? Maybe it's rare, but who would just make something like that up?

"The myths about increased cholesterol, heart problems, and other metabolic issues related to a vasectomy are really just myth."

Now I was getting a little worried. None of this stuff had even occurred to me before I came into this guy's office. Now he had my head filled with all kinds of horrifying images.

"You can even go back to normal sexual activity the following day, provided you're up for it," he said. "Just no Olympic-style mounts and dismounts for at least a week."

Does "normal sexual activity" generally constitute mounts and dismounts? Did I miss a memo? I mean, I made two babies so I know I'm doing something right, but I have no leotards, no hand chalk, and certainly no scorecards around when this kind of thing takes place.

"Now it's important to keep in mind," he warned, "that you may still be fertile for some time after the operation . . ."

Sounds like the opposite effect I'm going for, doc.

"So you'll want to perform a minimum of fifteen ejaculations alone or with protection before we check to make sure all your little swimmers are out of commission. I'll give you a jar to take home after the operation that you can use to bring a sample back to the lab for us to check out once you get to fifteen."

"You have to get the sample here pretty quickly after you produce it though, because those little buggers start to liquefy in about an hour or so."

No pressure there. Just goo in a cup, then race across town to let a team of strangers dig around in it, making sure you don't stop for coffee along the way.

"Sounds good," I lied, and walked back to my car wondering why I was talking about paying 900 bucks for a guy to hack away at my nuts.

I had to pay up front, in cash: no checks, no credit cards. Bills only. I felt a little like a Mafioso, coming in the morning of the deed and plopping an envelope full of hundreds on the counter. I might have made some joke to that effect, but I was too busy thinking about the procedure.

They called me back, had me strip from the waist-down, and "cover" myself with a giant napkin that was supposed to lend some sense of privacy.

"By the way," the nurse said, "that's one way glass, so no one can see in. But if you'd feel more comfortable, we can close the blinds."

"If someone can actually see in here and has the stomach to watch," I said, "they get what they deserve." She left me alone, my bare ass sliding down the sloped table covered with wax butcher paper. The bench was just long enough to support me to about my knees, and the raised back combined with sitting on wax paper made for an awkward situation. I tried to kind of pucker up my butt to grab hold of anything I could, but the only solution was putting my feet up on the corners, which stuck my bare ass straight out toward the door.

Then I waited. I know it was only ten minutes or so in human time, but my balls were sure it was an eternity.

You can still back out, they said to me. *I'm sure they'll give you your money back.*

I can't, balls. I promised Amy I'd do this.

But what did we ever do to you—aside from give you two great kids, which is what you wanted, right?

Yeah, thanks for that. But consider yourself retired.

What about condoms?

No chance, said the penis.

The doc finally came in, and I wasn't sure he remembered what he was there for. I expected him to be in scrubs or to at least have on a mask or something. But he was dressed more like he was headed to a business meeting. He even had his wristwatch on. It's not like I expected him to lose it inside my scrotum or anything, but it seemed an awfully casual approach to an event over which I had lost no few hours of sleep.

"I'm going to shave your scrotum before we start," he said, grabbing disposable razor from the tray next to him. "If I sewed a pubic hair up in your incision, you'd know, pronto."

"I would think so," I said, as he scraped at my sack with the razor. I was oddly impressed with how dexterous the guy was with a blade. I mean, it was a full-on dry shave, but he didn't knick the skin or anything. If you're going to have a guy fiddle with your hardware, better one who knows what he's doing, I say.

"Now we'll numb the area with Novocain," he grabbed a syringe. By then I had accepted that this guy was old-school enough that he was not likely to offer me a Valium or anything to calm me down, but now he had a needle in his hand and had yet to do anything to numb the particularly sensitive area he had in mind to poke with it.

Oh, hell no, said my nuts and started a full-on retreat.

And as you might expect, getting poked in the testicles several times with a needle is not the most comfortable sensation you can imagine. Thankfully, Novocain is fast-acting, so the sting went away within thirty seconds or so. In the meantime though, I had to hold tight to the sides of the table so I would not give into my reflexive impulse to whack him across the back of the head.

I guess everything relaxed down there after that because the left side went fast and pretty easy. I could feel some tugging up in my abdomen, but there was nothing I would consider to be overly painful. After about ten minutes or so, I had even gotten used to having a dude fondling my goodies, especially now that I couldn't feel it.

The right side was not so cooperative. It turns out, as the doctor later explained as he peeled me off the ceiling, that the second side often pulls back, to the point that the testicle is up inside the body when it gets wind of what's happening to its little buddy. This means that he's got to reach way up in there and do some pretty serious tugging to get at what he needs. Apparently, as I also learned, there are some nerves further up in there that don't benefit from the local anesthetic applied to the scrotum.

"Wow," I said, trying not to close my knees against his temples. "That was, um, unexpected."

"Sorry about that," he picked up his cauterizing gun. "Sometimes the second one's a little more stubborn. Tries to run and hide on you."

Oh, and in case you were curious, the smell of burning vas deferens is not particularly pleasant. I was hoping I'd be able to report something glibber about it smelling like chicken, but no deal. It smelled about how I thought burning balls might smell.

Before sewing me up, he left me with one final parting gift by grazing me with the cauterizing gun.

"Hey!" I squawked, "I think you burned me there."

"Hmm, yeah. A little bit there," he said nonchalantly. This is probably less than shocking, but there is nothing minor about any incident wherein your scrotum is burned with a hot iron. Maybe he thought it would be numb so he had some room for error.

Not so much.

He gave me a giant ice pack and a three-inch thick pad of gauze to stick in my shorts. He called it a "shock absorber."

"Make sure not to let your little ones hop on your lap for a few days," he said, handing me the container for my soon-to-be-spermless sample. "Take some Tylenol if it starts to hurt and try to stay off your feet for about twelve hours."

Three days later, things are starting to look much more normal down there. Mattias has been very curious about my progress and he understands that a leap on the lap will be cause for immediate grounding. I'm back to being able to pick up Zoe, which is nice, and I can help with most of my basic duties around the house.

As for the whole sex-the-next-day thing, that didn't happen.

I have to admit that the long-term prospect of pressure-free intimacy for the rest of my life feels pretty good, and I'm glad to take my share of the responsibility for our family planning. I just hope some day that my boys will find it in their little hearts to forgive me. It's been a good run, fellas, but your work here is officially done.